Digital Health, AI and Generative AI in Healthcare

Terry Adirim
Editor

Digital Health, AI and Generative AI in Healthcare

A Concise, Practical Guide for Clinicians

Springer

Editor
Terry Adirim
Departments of Pediatrics
and Preventive Medicine and Biostatistics
Uniformed Services
University of the Health Sciences
Bethesda, MD, USA

ISBN 978-3-031-83525-4 ISBN 978-3-031-83526-1 (eBook)
https://doi.org/10.1007/978-3-031-83526-1

This Springer imprint is published by the registered company Springer Nature Switzerland AG
The registered company address is: Gewerbestrasse 11, 6330 Cham, Switzerland

Introduction

Over 30 years ago, when I entered medical school, patient care always took place in a medical office or hospital, the visit documented on paper, retrieving medical records involved submitting a paper request at the medical records department (with the medical student picking it up), retrieving scientific journal articles consisted of accessing paper index medicus listings published monthly, and to access the actual publications, one had to photocopy the article directly from the paper version of the journal. So much has changed in medicine since with the rise of electronic medical records, the evolution of electronic search engines such as NIH's PubMed, electronic access to scientific journals, and rapid innovations in digital health technologies. I have been privileged to practice during the 1990s and 2000s where I experienced a time of rapid advancements in how healthcare was documented, delivered, and researched. Further acceleration occurred during the COVID-19 pandemic, out of necessity, with the widespread use of telehealth and remote monitoring technologies. With the introduction of generative AI, including the release of Open AI's ChatGPT in 2022, we are entering a new age of rapid advancements in technology that will again significantly change the way we practice medicine, how we operate our healthcare institutions, and how we conduct research.

Medical schools, medical training programs, and other health education institutions must undertake a key role in developing AI literacy for clinicians across the spectrum of medical education and training that includes all health professions. AI literacy should be incorporated within medical school curriculums as a core competency as well as into graduate medical education training programs and continuing medical education courses. Medical professionals need a fundamental understanding of AI, including a basic understanding of algorithms, machine learning, large language models, and natural language processing, as well as an awareness of how AI is currently being used in healthcare. Perhaps more critically, clinicians must understand the limits and pitfalls of AI. Moreover, clinicians will need an understanding of the ethical and legal issues associated with the use of AI, such as the current and evolving regulatory landscape, rules on data privacy, the potential overt and implicit biases of AI outputs, and requirements for transparency.

Additionally, AI technologies will change how medical school curriculums are delivered and student competencies assessed. This transformation has already started, driven in part by the COVID-19 pandemic that required medical schools to deliver their didactic curriculums virtually. Also, consider that the amount of medical data available in the 1990s compared to today has increased exponentially due to the digitation of medical records and the rise of data-generating technologies. In the 1990s, medical knowledge was estimated to double approximately every 7–10 years as opposed to current estimates of medical knowledge doubling every 73–120 days. Accessing this vastly larger, more complex, and every growing store of information is easier now than when I was a medical student. This vast amount of information cannot be memorized. Therefore, medical educators need to consider how and what medical information is taught to students during formal instruction, and importantly how to access information when it is needed. Educators must be prepared for AI-powered programs that will be used to assess students and trainees not just within educational institutions but also for the purpose of licensure and board certification.

These emerging technologies will require not only reimagining the learning experience for students but also require providing education in the basics of health informatics, data analytics, and the use of digital technologies. This book provides a foundation for all medical professionals and is well suited to serve as a resource for all healthcare profession students and medical professionals interested in understanding AI. This book would not be possible without the expertise and thoughtful guidance of the contributing authors. Thank you to these leaders in their fields for sharing their expertise and to the inspiring founders of healthcare startups advancing the use of AI in healthcare who I have met as I worked on this book.

Bethesda, MD, USA Terry Adirim

Contents

Contributors

Alyssa Abo Impact1 at Stanford Mussallem Center for Biodesign, Stanford Medicine, Stanford, CA, USA

Terry Adirim Departments of Pediatrics and Preventive Medicine and Biostatistics, Uniformed Services University of the Health Sciences, Bethesda, MD, USA

Karen Blades WhirlyBee Consulting, Washington, DC, USA

Thomas J. Cantilina Formerly Department of Defense, Defense Health Agency, Falls Church, VA, USA

David Carnahan Amazon Web Services, Worldwide Public Sector, San Antonio, TX, USA

Todd P. Chang Department of Pediatrics, Division of Emergency Medicine & Transport, Keck School of Medicine of USC, Los Angeles, CA, USA

Taylor Freeburg Department of Pediatrics, Children's Hospital Los Angeles, Los Angeles, CA, USA

Karen Habercoss The University of Chicago Medicine, Chicago, IL, USA

Shannon Lantzy Shannon Lantzy, LLC, Silver Spring, MD, USA

Ranit Mishori Georgetown University School of Medicine, Washington, DC, USA

Amy Molten Department of Pediatrics, Tufts Medical Center, Boston, MA, USA

Rashmi Rao University of Washington, Engineering Innovation in Health (EIH), Sammamish, WA, USA

Holly Urban Wolters Kluwer Health, Waltham, MA, USA

Part I
Foundations of Digital Health and AI

Chapter 1
The History of Digital Health and Artificial Intelligence

Terry Adirim

Introduction

As adoption of new technologies accelerates, it is useful to understand how we have arrived to this point of major transformation in the delivery of health care. The evolution of digital health and artificial intelligence (AI) has been enabled by the integration of health information technology (IT), wearables, telehealth, and personalized medicine as well as the accumulation of large amounts of data. The adoption of technologies has accelerated in recent years due to federal programs that incentivized and facilitated the adoption of electronic health records and was given a boost during the COVID-19 pandemic when most healthcare systems and practices implemented virtual health to maintain safe medical encounters with patients. AI has gone from theoretical concepts to the development of generative models representing a significant trajectory in computational and cognitive science over the last decade. Generative AI has been enabled by large amounts of data available on the internet. This confluence of advances in digital tools, AI and availability of data has the potential to substantially change how we practice medicine. These advances are built upon advances and discoveries over many decades. In recognition of the impact on society AI is and will have, the 2024 Nobel Prize in Physics was awarded to two computer scientists, John J. Hopfield and Geoffrey E. Hinton for their foundational work in neural networks performed in the 1980s [1]. These scientists' early work laid the foundation for machine learning that has made current generative AI possible.

T. Adirim (✉)
Departments of Pediatrics and Preventive Medicine and Biostatistics,
Uniformed Services University of the Health Sciences, Bethesda, MD, USA

T. Adirim (ed.), *Digital Health, AI and Generative AI in Healthcare*,
https://doi.org/10.1007/978-3-031-83526-1_1

The History of Digital Health

The concept of digital health has evolved significantly over the past few decades, transitioning from basic digitization efforts in healthcare to sophisticated platforms and tools that provide deep insights intended to improve healthcare outcomes. At its core, digital health encompasses a wide range of technologies including, but not limited to, electronic health records (EHRs), telehealth, mobile health (mHealth), wearable devices, and personalized medicine.

The history of digital health can be traced back to the first attempts at digitizing health records in the late twentieth century. The development of electronic health records (EHRs) in the 1960s and 1970s marked the beginning of this journey, aiming to improve the accessibility and quality of patient information [2]. EHRs laid the groundwork for a more systematic approach to health data management, setting the stage for future innovations in digital health.

Telehealth emerged as a critical component of digital health by using telecommunications technology to provide healthcare services remotely. Telehealth has its origins as early as the early twentieth century, but it was not until the 1960s and 1970s that significant advancements were made, facilitated by improvements in telecommunications technology [3]. The introduction of the internet and mobile technology further accelerated the development of telehealth, making it a key element in addressing issues of accessibility and cost in healthcare.

The proliferation of smartphones and wearable technology in the early twenty-first century marked a significant milestone in the evolution of digital health. Mobile health (mHealth) applications and wearable devices have changed the way health data can be collected, monitored, and analyzed, offering unprecedented opportunities for personalized health management and preventive care [4]. These technologies have enabled continuous health monitoring outside traditional healthcare settings, empowering patients and healthcare providers with real-time data and insights. Moreover, reliable telehealth technologies have in recent years enabled a proliferation of companies that deliver therapeutics virtually such as antivirals during the COVID-19 pandemic and GLP-1 agonist medications more recently.

The History and Evolution of Artificial Intelligence

Generative AI was introduced in the 1960s through chatbots but it was not until 2014 with the development of generative adversarial networks, otherwise known as GANs, that generative AI could begin to show its potential in producing authentic audio and images [5]. Soon after, companies such as Google and Open AI developed precursors to public generative AI tools.

AI begins in an environment of intellectual curiosity and quest to determine if machines could mimic or surpass human intelligence. The foundations of AI are deeply rooted in mathematics, logic, philosophy, and computer science, creating a multidisciplinary approach to tackling the complexities of intelligent behavior.

Before the invention of digital computers, the concept of "artificial intelligence" was a product of imagination, Philosophers and mathematicians pondered the nature of thought and the possibility of creating artificial minds. The groundwork for AI was laid by pioneers such as George Boole and Gottlob Frege, who developed the formal logical systems in the nineteenth and early twentieth centuries, forming the basis for computational logic [6]. It was Alan Turing, a British mathematician and logician, who made a groundbreaking contribution to the development of AI in his 1950 paper, "Computing Machinery and Intelligence" where he proposed the idea that machines could be made to simulate human intelligence, introducing the famous Turing Test as a criterion for intelligence in machines [7]. Turing's work not only posed the fundamental question, "Can machines think?" but also provided a conceptual framework for future AI research.

The formal birth of AI as a distinct field of study is often traced back to the Dartmouth Conference of 1956. The proposal for this conference stated that "every aspect of learning or any other feature of intelligence can in principle be so precisely described that a machine can be made to simulate it [8]. This conference marked the coining of the term "Artificial Intelligence" and set the stage for decades of research, exploration, and debate within the field.

In the early years, AI research was dominated by the symbolic approach, which focused on encoding knowledge into logical rules and manipulating these rules to achieve intelligent behavior. This approach was underpinned by the belief that intelligence arises from the ability to use symbols to represent the world and to perform reasoning tasks with these symbols. Pioneering systems demonstrated the potential of symbolic AI in understanding natural language and engaging in simple forms of human-computer interaction [9]. At the same time, another approach was being developed called connectionism, or the study of neural networks. Inspired by the structure and function of the human brain, this approach sought to create artificial intelligence through interconnected networks of simple units (neurons) that could learn from experience. While initially overshadowed by the symbolic approach, interest in neural networks surged in the 1980s with the development of algorithms for training multi-layer perceptrons (a neural network unit), leading to what is now known as deep learning [10].

The initial decades following AI's conception were marked by ambitious projects. Researchers developed systems that could solve algebra problems, prove theorems, and understand natural language to a limited extent. These early successes, however, were soon tempered by the realization that scaling these systems to handle real-world complexity was not as straightforward as initially conceived. The limitations of early AI were highlighted in the Lighthill Report (1973), which criticized the oversold promises of AI [11].

The Evolution of AI

The resurgence of neural networks in the late twentieth and early twenty-first centuries has been critical in the evolution of AI. This resurgence occurred due to the development of deep learning techniques, which utilized layered architectures of neural networks to learn hierarchical representations of data. This approach allowed for significant advances in fields such as computer vision, natural language processing, and speech recognition. A pivotal moment in the advancement of AI occurred in 2016 when DeepMind's AlphaGo beat the world champion Go player, a feat that demonstrated the potential of deep learning models to undertake complex strategic challenges [12].

The growth of digital data and the parallel increase in computational power have been crucial drivers of AI's recent advancements. The availability of large datasets has enabled the training of more sophisticated and accurate models, while advances in hardware, particularly GPUs, have drastically reduced the time required to train such models. This synergy between data availability and computational power has accelerated the pace of innovation in AI, making technologies like autonomous vehicles and real-time language translation a reality.

The History of Machine Learning, Deep Learning and Big Data

Machine learning is a subset of AI that focuses on the development of algorithms that can learn from and make predictions or decisions based on data. This shift towards machine learning was fueled by the realization that manually programming complex behaviors and knowledge into AI systems was impractical and limiting. Pioneers in machine learning such as 2024 Nobel Prize recipients John Hopfield and Georffrey Hinton who laid the foundational theories for neural networks and deep learning, demonstrated that machines could learn complex representations and perform tasks like object recognition, language translation, and even game playing at or above human levels [13].

Deep learning, a subset of machine learning that is characterized by deep neural networks with many layers, emerged as a powerful tool for AI, enabling significant advancements in processing images, sound, and text data. The success of deep learning models in various competitions such as the ImageNet Large Scale Visual Recognition Challenge highlighted their potential and spurred increased investment and interest in AI research [14].

The phrase "big data" refers to datasets that are too large or complex to be dealt with by traditional data-processing application software. The digital age has seen an explosion in the amount and variety of data available, driven by the widespread adoption of the internet, social media, mobile devices, and the Internet of Things (IoT). This abundance of data has been a crucial factor in the rise of machine learning, providing the raw material needed to train increasingly sophisticated models. Big data has not only provided the fuel for machine learning but has also raised new challenges and opportunities in data storage, processing, and analysis. Techniques and infrastructures such as distributed computing, cloud services, and advanced data analytics have been developed to manage the scale and complexity of big data [15].

The Progression to Generative Artificial Intelligence

The latest in the evolution of Artificial Intelligence (AI) is the rise of generative artificial intelligence (gen AI), a type of AI that not only understands and analyzes data but also creates and generates new content. This capability represents a significant leap from traditional AI systems, enabling machines to design images, write text, and compose music that are indistinguishable from—or even potentially surpass—the creations of humans. The development of generative AI models, such as Generative Adversarial Networks (GANs) and Variational Autoencoders (VAEs), has led to a new era in AI, where the creative and generative capacities of machines open unprecedented possibilities. Introduced in 2014, GANs) represent a breakthrough in the field of gen AI [16]. A GAN consists of two neural networks—the generator and the discriminator—trained simultaneously through adversarial processes. The generator creates data resembling the training set, while the discriminator evaluates its authenticity. This competition drives the generator to produce increasingly realistic data, leading to more precise results in image generation, photo-realistic rendering, and even video synthesis. GANs have revolutionized fields such as computer graphics, fashion, and design, demonstrating the creative potential of AI.

Another term, Variational Autoencoders, provides another approach to generative modeling and was only recently reported in 2013 [17]. VAEs are designed to encode input data into a lower-dimensional space and then reconstruct it, with the aim of learning the probability distribution of the data. This mechanism enables VAEs to generate new data points with similar properties to those in the training set. VAEs have been particularly influential in generating complex data structures such as faces, voices, and even molecular structures, contributing to advancements in synthetic biology, chemistry, and personalized media.

Gen AI has potential to provide great improvements across various sectors including healthcare. In creative industries, artists and designers leverage these technologies to explore new forms of expression and creativity. In the field of healthcare, generative models have the potential to improve the delivery of care, support clinicians in their work, aid in drug discovery and advance the creation of personalized medicine. Furthermore, gen AI has a potential role in enhancing data privacy through synthetic data generation, allowing the development and testing of AI systems without compromising sensitive information (Table 1.1).

Table 1.1 Timeline of events leading to generative AI

Year	Event
1932	Georges Artsrouni invents a machine he reportedly called the "mechanical brain" to translate between languages on a mechanical computer encoded onto punch cards.
1957	Linguist Noam Chomsky publishes Syntactic Structures, paper that describes grammatical rules for parsing and generating natural language sentences.
1966	MIT professor Joseph Weizenbaum creates the first chatbot, Eliza, which simulates conversations with a psychotherapist.
1968	Computer science professor Terry Winograd creates the first multimodal AI (SHRDLU) that manipulates and reasons out a world of blocks according to instructions from a user.
1980	Michael Toy and Glenn Wichman develop the Unix-based game Rogue that uses procedural content generation to dynamically generate new game levels.
1985	Computer scientist and philosopher Judea Pearl introduces Bayesian networks causal analysis, which provides statistical techniques for representing uncertainty that leads to methods for generating content in a specific style, tone, or length.
1986	Michael Irwin Jordan lays the foundation for the modern use of recurrent neural networks (RNNs) with the publication of Serial order: a parallel distributed processing approach.
1989	Yann LeCun, Yoshua Bengio, and Patrick Haffner demonstrate how convolutional neural networks (CNNs) can be used to recognize images.
2000	Researchers from the University of Montreal publish A Neural Probabilistic Language Model, which suggests a method to model language using feed-forward neural networks.
2006	Data scientist Fei-Fei Li sets up the ImageNet database, which provides the foundation for visual object recognition.
2011	Apple releases Siri, a voice-powered personal assistant that generates responses and takes actions in response to spoken requests.
2012	Alex Krizhevsky designs the AlexNet CNN architecture, pioneering a new way of automatically training neural networks that take advantage of recent GPU advances.
2013	Google researcher Tomas Mikolov introduces word2vec that identifies semantic relationships between words automatically.
2014	• Research scientist Ian Goodfellow develops generative adversarial networks (GANs) that pit two neural networks against each other to generate increasingly realistic content. • Diederik Kingma and Max Welling introduce variational autoencoders to generate images, videos, and text.
2015	Stanford researchers publish work on diffusion models in the paper Deep Unsupervised Learning using Nonequilibrium Thermodynamics. The technique provides a way to reverse-engineer the process of adding noise to a final image.
2017	Google researchers develop the concept of transformers in the seminal paper Attention is all you need, inspiring subsequent research into tools that could automatically parse unlabeled text into large language models (LLMs).
2018	• Google researchers implement transformers into BERT, which is trained on more than 3.3 billion words and can automatically learn the relationship between words in sentences, paragraphs, and even books to predict the meaning of text. • Google DeepMind researchers developed AlphaFold for predicting protein structures, laying the foundation for generative AI applications in medical research, drug development, and chemistry. • OpenAI releases GPT (Generative Pre-trained Transformer). Trained on about 40 gigabytes of data and consisting of 117 million parameters, GPT paves the way for subsequent LLMs in content generation, chatbots, and language translation.

(continued)

Table 1.1 (continued)

Year	Event
2021	OpenAI introduces DALL·E, which can generate images from text prompts. DALL-E is a combination of WALL-E, the name of a fictional robot, and the artist Salvador Dali.
2022	OpenAI releases ChatGPT in November that provides a chat-based interface to its GPT 3.5 LLM. Within two months, there are over 100 million users, representing the fastest-ever consumer adoption of a service.
2023	Microsoft integrates a version of ChatGPT into its Bing search engine. Google quickly followed with plans to release the Bard chat service based on its Lamda engine. Controversy over detecting AI-generated content increases.
2024	John J. Hopfield and Geoffrey E. Hinton are awarded the Nobel Prize in Physicians "for foundational discoveries and inventions that enable machine learning with artificial neural networks" (Nobel press release)

Information Sources for the Table:
History of generative AI innovations spans 9 decades—TechTarget, https://www.techtarget.com/searchenterpriseai/tip/History-of-generative-AI-innovations-spans-9-decades
What is generative AI? Definition, models, and use cases—WalkMe Blog, https://www.walkme.com/blog/what-is-generative-ai/
AI is transforming the data center—Principal Financial Group, https://brandassets.principal.com/m/1a67963b880ada3f/original/Principal-Real-Estate-AI-is-transforming-the-data-center.pdf
History and evolution of machine learning: A timeline—TechTarget, https://www.techtarget.com/whatis/A-Timeline-of-Machine-Learning-History
Generative Pre-trained Transformer (GPT) in AI/ML-Enabled Medtech Industry, https://marketingable.mphasis.com/content/dam/mphasis-com/global/en/home/industries/medtech-page/Mphasis-Whitepaper-Impact-of-GPT-in-AI-ML-enabled-MedTech-Industry.pdf
The Nobel Prize in Physics 2024—Press Release. NobelPrize.org. Published October 8, 2024. Accessed October 15, 2024. https://www.nobelprize.org/prizes/physics/2024/press-release/

Conclusion

The evolution of digital and AI technology has taken place over many decades leading to new technologies that have the potential to change how and where we practice medicine. Understanding the technology and its potential and pitfalls is critical for all clinicians.

References

1. The Nobel Prize in Physics 2024—Press Release. NobelPrize.org. Published October 8, 2024. https://www.nobelprize.org/prizes/physics/2024/press-release/. Accessed 15 Oct 2024.
2. Evans RS. Electronic health records: then, now, and in the future. Yearb Med Inform. 2016;Suppl 1(Suppl 1):S48–61.
3. Bashshur RL, Shannon GW. History of telemedicine: evolution, context, and transformation. New Rochelle: Mary Ann Liebert, Inc.; 2009.
4. Free C, Phillips G, Watson L, Galli L, Felix L, Edwards P, Patel V, Haines A. The effectiveness of mobile-health technologies to improve health care service delivery processes: a systematic review and meta-analysis. PLoS Med. 2013;10(1):e1001363.

5. Lawton G. What is generative AI? Everything you need to know. Tech Target. https://www.techtarget.com/searchenterpriseai/definition/generative-AI#:~:text=Generative%20AI%20was%20introduced%20in,and%20audio%20of%20real%20people. Site Updated April, 2024. Accessed 1 June 2024.
6. Boole G. An investigation of the laws of thought: on which are founded the mathematical theories of logic and probabilities. Cambridge: Cambridge University Press; 2009. First published in 1854.
7. Turing AM. Computing machinery and intelligence. Mind. 1950;LIX(236):433–60.
8. McCarthy J, Minsky ML, Rochester N, Shannon CE. A proposal for the Dartmouth summer research project on artificial intelligence; 1956.
9. Winograd T. Understanding natural language. Cogn Psychol. 1972;3(1):1–191.
10. Rumelhart D, Hinton G, Williams R. Learning representations by back-propagating errors. Nature. 1986;323:533–6.
11. Lighthill J. Artificial intelligence: a general survey. In: Artificial intelligence: a paper symposium; 1973.
12. Silver D, Huang A, Maddison CJ, et al. Mastering the game of Go with deep neural networks and tree search. Nature. 2016;529(7587):484–9.
13. LeCun Y, Bengio Y, Hinton G. Deep learning. Nature. 2015;521(7553):436–44.
14. Russakovsky O, Deng J, Su H, et al. ImageNet large scale visual recognition challenge. Int J Comput Vis. 2015;115(3):211–52.
15. Mayer-Schönberger V, Cukier K. Big data: a revolution that Will transform how we live, work, and think. Boston: Houghton Mifflin Harcourt; 2013.
16. Goodfellow I, Pouget-Abadie J, Mirza M, et al. Generative adversarial nets. In: Advances in neural information processing systems. Cambridge, MA: MIT Press; 2014. p. 2672–80.
17. Kingma DP, Welling M. Auto-encoding variational Bayes. In: International conference on learning representations; 2013.

Chapter 2
Digital Health Technologies: Virtual Health and Remote Patient Monitoring

Terry Adirim

Introduction

The healthcare landscape is rapidly evolving, driven by technological advancements and changing patient needs. Among these advancements, virtual health technologies, such as telehealth and remote monitoring, have emerged as pivotal components of modern healthcare delivery. These technologies have revolutionized patient care by enabling remote consultations, more frequent monitoring, and dissemination of hospital-at-home programs. This chapter explores virtual health technologies' evolution, benefits, challenges, and future prospects.

Evolution of Virtual Health Technologies

The Rise of Telehealth

Telehealth, the delivery of healthcare services through telecommunication technologies, has roots in the early twentieth century but gained significant momentum in the late twentieth and early twenty-first centuries. Initially, telehealth was primarily used for consultations between healthcare providers in remote areas. However, with advancements in internet connectivity, mobile technology, and digital health tools, telehealth has expanded to include a wide range of services such as remote patient consultations, telepsychiatry, teledermatology, digital therapeutics (on-line ordering and dispensing of medications), and other use cases.

T. Adirim (✉)
Departments of Pediatrics and Preventive Medicine and Biostatistics,
Uniformed Services University of the Health Sciences, Bethesda, MD, USA

T. Adirim (ed.), *Digital Health, AI and Generative AI in Healthcare*,
https://doi.org/10.1007/978-3-031-83526-1_2

Emergence of Remote Monitoring Technologies

Remote monitoring technologies have developed alongside telehealth, driven by the need for more frequent patient care outside traditional healthcare settings. Remote patient monitoring (RPM) involves using digital devices to collect and transmit patient data, such as vital signs, from a patient's home to healthcare providers [1]. This technology has enabled the development of programs like hospital-at-home, where patients receive hospital-level care in the comfort of their homes [2].

Telehealth: Transforming Healthcare Delivery

The Scope of Telehealth

Telehealth encompasses various services, including real-time video consultations, store-and-forward technologies for transmitting medical data, remote patient monitoring, and mobile health (mHealth) applications. The COVID-19 pandemic significantly accelerated the adoption of telehealth, making it a mainstream modality for delivering healthcare [3]. During the pandemic, the Centers for Medicare and Medicaid Services provided waivers and flexibilities during the COVID-19 public health emergency that facilitated expansion of telehealth healthcare delivery. Telehealth provided a safe and effective way for patients to access healthcare services while minimizing the risk of virus transmission [4, 5]. Telehealth use will continue to expand, especially to support access to care in resource-limited care environments like rural, remote, and disaster settings [6].

Benefits of Telehealth

Telehealth expands access to care, bridging the gap between patients and healthcare providers, particularly in rural and underserved areas where access to healthcare facilities may be limited. Patients can now receive timely medical consultations without the need for long-distance travel.

Telehealth offers convenience for both patients and providers. Patients can schedule appointments and receive care from the comfort of their homes, while providers can manage their schedules more flexibly. Additionally, telehealth can reduce healthcare costs by minimizing the need for physical infrastructure, reducing hospital readmissions, and lowering patient transportation costs. Another benefit for patients and clinicians is that telehealth programs facilitate continuous monitoring and follow-up, improving chronic disease management and reducing the risk of complications.

Challenges and Barriers to Telehealth Adoption

Despite the widespread availability of telehealth technologies, limited internet access, especially in rural areas, and patient technological literacy can hinder telehealth adoption. The regulatory landscape for telehealth is complex and varies by region. Reimbursement policies for telehealth services are still evolving, creating uncertainty for healthcare providers and patients.

The use of telecommunication technologies in healthcare raises concerns about data privacy and security. Ensuring the confidentiality of patient information during telehealth consultations is critical.

While telehealth offers many benefits, it may also reduce the personal interaction between patients and providers, potentially impacting the quality of and satisfaction with care. Building trust and maintaining effective communication in a virtual setting is challenging. Therefore, virtual health should not be a substitute for in person care, but rather should serve as a support to the patient and provider relationship.

Remote Patient Monitoring: Enhancing Patient Care Beyond Hospital Walls

The Role of Remote Monitoring Technologies

Remote patient monitoring (RPM) technologies have transformed healthcare delivery by allowing continuous monitoring of patients' health conditions outside of traditional healthcare settings. RPM devices collect and transmit data such as heart rate, blood pressure, glucose levels, and oxygen saturation to healthcare providers, enabling real-time monitoring and early intervention.

Hospital-at-Home Programs

Hospital-at-home programs are an emerging innovative application of RPM technologies, allowing patients to receive hospital-level care in their homes [5]. These programs are particularly beneficial for patients with chronic conditions, those with post-operative care needs, or those requiring palliative care, but these programs have also been used to reduce emergency room overcrowding and hospital admissions. Hospital-at-home programs reduce the burden on hospitals, can potentially lower healthcare costs, and improve patient satisfaction by allowing patients to recover in a familiar environment [5, 7, 8].

Benefits of Remote Monitoring

RPM technologies have the potential to support the early detection of potential health issues, allowing for timely interventions and reducing the risk of complications. RPM allows for continuous monitoring of patients' health conditions that can prevent hospital readmissions by managing symptoms and providing care before conditions worsen.

Additionally, RPM empowers patients to actively manage their health by providing real-time data and insights into their health status. Since RPM reduces the need for in-person visits, hospital stays, and emergency room visits, there is the potential for significant cost savings for patients and healthcare providers.

Challenges in Implementing Remote Monitoring

Health systems and institutions often face challenges facilitating patients' and providers' adoption of new technologies. Like telehealth, the successful implementation of RPM requires patients to have access to reliable technology and internet connectivity. Patients must also be trained to use these devices effectively.

Data management and integration are significant challenges for healthcare institutions establishing these programs. The vast amount of data generated by RPM devices presents challenges in data management, integration, and analysis. Healthcare providers need efficient systems to manage and interpret this data or risk that patient collected data will go unused.

The healthcare regulatory landscape is complex and ever-changing, posing challenges to these programs. The reimbursement policies for RPM services are still evolving, with variations in coverage and payment models. Additionally, the regulatory framework for RPM is complex and varies by region. Moreover, ensuring patient engagement and adherence to RPM protocols is critical for the success of remote monitoring programs. Patients must be motivated and supported to use these technologies consistently.

Virtual Health Use Case for Chronic Disease Management

An example of a common remote monitoring program that has been shown to benefit patients includes remote monitoring for patients with Congestive Heart Failure (CHF) as a tool to prevent exacerbations. These programs include providing devices and equipment to patients' homes, such as blood pressure monitors, weight scales, and pulse oximeters that are Bluetooth or cellular connective enabled. These devices automatically transmit data to a cloud-based platform. Some programs might include wearable devices that monitor heart rate, oxygen saturation, physical activity levels, and EKG patterns. The data collected can be displayed on a dashboard accessible by the patient's provider, who can monitor these clinical parameters in real-time.

These systems include algorithms that analyze trends and identify potential health concerns, such as a sudden increase in weight that could be due to fluid retention or new heart arrhythmias, sending alerts to the patient's healthcare team. The team reviews the data and can provide any needed follow-up, such as medication adjustments, diet modification, or additional tests. Additionally, virtual consultations or in-person visits can be scheduled at home if needed, especially for older, more medically fragile patients for whom travel can be challenging. These platforms also benefit from providing educational content to patients, such as diet recommendations, exercise tips, and how to take medications. For the clinicians who care for these patients, these tools provide trends and regular reports on clinical status that can be incorporated into the patient's electronic health record, which is useful in guiding care. The American Medical Association provides a playbook on how to establish these programs [7]. Importantly, these programs have been shown to reduce hospital readmissions [8], improve clinical outcomes and quality of life [9], provide cost savings [10, 11], and promote patient engagement and self-management [12, 13].

Other Current and Emerging Uses of Virtual Consultation and Digital Health Services

Teleradiology

Teleradiology is a branch of telemedicine that has been in use in the United States since the 1980s and advanced significantly in the 1990s and 2000s as digital imaging technologies matured and internet connectivity became faster, leading to Picture Archiving and Communication Systems (PACS). It involves the electronic transmission of radiological images, such as X-rays, CT scans, MRIs, and ultrasounds, from one location to another for interpretation and consultation. This technology enables radiologists to provide diagnostic services remotely, allowing healthcare facilities to offer 24/7 radiology support, even in locations where in-person radiologist services are not readily available [14].

The primary advantage of teleradiology lies in its ability to bridge the gap in radiological services, especially in rural or underserved areas. Many healthcare facilities, such as small hospitals, clinics, and imaging centers, may not have access to full-time radiologists. Teleradiology connects these facilities to a network of radiologists who can provide expert interpretation of imaging studies, often in real-time. This rapid access to specialist expertise enhances patient care by speeding up diagnosis and treatment. For example, a radiologist in a different city or country can promptly review emergency cases like trauma injuries or acute neurological conditions, offering timely input that can be crucial for patient outcomes [15].

Teleradiology services typically use secure, encrypted networks to transmit images and patient information, complying with health privacy laws such as the Health Insurance Portability and Accountability Act (HIPAA) in the United States [16]. PACS systems efficiently store and transmit digital medical images. Radiologists can access these systems via computers, tablets, or smartphones, allowing them to work remotely while maintaining high diagnostic accuracy. Some advanced teleradiology platforms even utilize artificial intelligence (AI) to assist with preliminary reads and triaging cases, which further optimizes the workflow and speeds up the diagnostic process.

Teleradiology improves access to radiology services and enhances workflow efficiency for healthcare facilities. By offloading image interpretation to remote radiologists, in-house clinicians can focus more on patient care. Additionally, access to a broader network of radiologists allows facilities to match cases to specialists with specific expertise in musculoskeletal, pediatric, or neuroradiology. This specialization can lead to more accurate interpretations and improved patient outcomes.

However, teleradiology also faces challenges. One primary concern is ensuring the security and confidentiality of patient data during electronic transmission. High-quality image resolution and reliable internet connections are essential to maintain diagnostic accuracy, as poor-quality images can lead to misinterpretation [17]. Furthermore, differences in medical licensing and regulations across states and countries can complicate the provision of teleradiology services. Despite these challenges, the use of teleradiology is expanding, driven by advancements in digital imaging technology, secure communication networks, and the growing demand for radiological services. As healthcare systems evolve, teleradiology is expected to play an increasingly vital role in delivering high-quality, efficient, and accessible diagnostic care.

Teledermatology

Teledermatology provides dermatological care through digital communication technologies using high-resolution images and video consultations to diagnose, monitor, and treat various skin conditions remotely [18]. By facilitating virtual consultations between patients and dermatologists, teledermatology addresses common barriers to dermatological care, such as long wait times for appointments and the limited availability of specialists in rural or underserved areas [19].

There are two primary modes of teledermatology: store-and-forward and real-time (live interactive). In the store-and-forward model, patients or healthcare providers capture and send images of skin lesions, rashes, and other dermatological concerns with the relevant medical history to a dermatologist for review [18]. The dermatologist then examines the images, provides a diagnosis, and suggests a treatment plan. This asynchronous approach allows dermatologists to review cases at their convenience, making it an efficient way to manage non-urgent dermatological conditions. The real-time or live interactive mode involves video consultations, where patients and dermatologists engage in a virtual face-to-face meeting. This method is advantageous for cases where direct interaction, visual assessment, and real-time discussion of symptoms are necessary.

Teledermatology has improved access to care, especially for patients in remote or underserved areas who might otherwise have to travel long distances to see a specialist. It also facilitates quicker diagnoses and management of skin conditions, reducing the need for in-person visits [19]. For example, patients with chronic skin diseases, such as psoriasis or eczema, can benefit from regular follow-up through teledermatology, allowing for timely adjustments to their treatment plans. Additionally, teledermatology can be lifesaving in cases of suspected skin cancers, such as melanoma, where early detection and intervention are critical.

However, the success of teledermatology depends on the quality of images captured and transmitted [20]. High-resolution cameras and appropriate lighting are crucial for accurately depicting skin lesions. Patient education on taking proper images is often necessary to ensure the dermatologist can accurately assess. Despite limitations, such as the inability to perform in-person procedures like biopsies, teledermatology has proven effective in many situations. Advances in artificial intelligence (AI) and machine learning are also enhancing teledermatology by providing automated image analysis to assist in the diagnosis of common skin conditions [21].

Teledermatology is increasingly integrated into routine dermatological practice, particularly in healthcare systems and clinics serving large or geographically dispersed patient populations. During the COVID-19 pandemic, the use of teledermatology expanded significantly as healthcare providers sought to minimize in-person contact while continuing to provide essential care [22]. This experience has demonstrated teledermatology's potential to enhance healthcare delivery and has accelerated its adoption as a valuable component of comprehensive dermatological care.

Telepsychiatry

Telepsychiatry (also Tele behavioral health) involves delivering psychiatric care and mental health services through telecommunications technology. It allows psychiatrists, psychologists, therapists, and other mental health professionals to conduct consultations, evaluations, therapy sessions, medication management, and follow-up sessions remotely. Telepsychiatry typically uses video conferencing as its primary medium, though other forms, such as phone calls, text messaging, and email, are also used for various aspects of mental health care. This method has become increasingly popular due to the flexibility and convenience it offers to providers and patients.

One of the significant benefits of telepsychiatry is improved access to mental health care, especially for individuals in rural or underserved areas where mental health professionals may be scarce [23]. Patients in these regions often face long travel distances, wait times, and limited appointment availability when seeking traditional in-person services. Telepsychiatry helps bridge this gap by providing timely access to care, which is crucial for patients with acute mental health conditions, including those experiencing anxiety, depression, or substance use disorders. Additionally, telepsychiatry can be beneficial for those with mobility issues, chronic physical illnesses, or time constraints that make regular in-person visits challenging [24].

Telepsychiatry also promotes continuity of care by allowing patients to maintain regular contact with their mental health providers, reducing the likelihood of missed appointments. This ongoing communication is vital for monitoring the patient's progress, adjusting treatment plans, and ensuring medication adherence. Patients often report feeling more comfortable and at ease in their own environment, which can potentially facilitate more open communication and engagement during therapy sessions. For healthcare systems and providers, telepsychiatry can be a cost-effective way to extend mental health services without additional physical infrastructure, thus helping to manage provider shortages [25].

Despite these advantages, telepsychiatry has several pitfalls. One primary concern is the potential for compromised confidentiality and privacy. The transmission of sensitive patient information over electronic communication platforms carries the risk of data breaches or unauthorized access if improperly secured [26]. Telepsychiatry services must adhere to privacy laws such as the Health Insurance Portability and Accountability Act (HIPAA) to protect patient information. In addition, technological challenges, including poor internet connectivity, may lead to interruptions during sessions and affect the quality of communication between the provider and the patient [27]. This issue is particularly relevant in rural or low-income areas where access to high-speed internet and appropriate devices may be limited.

Another potential drawback is the limited ability to perform physical assessments. While psychiatric evaluations primarily rely on verbal and behavioral cues, certain aspects of mental health care, such as assessing physical signs of substance withdrawal or side effects of medications, are harder to evaluate through a screen. There is also the challenge of managing emergencies remotely. Providers may face difficulties intervening in crises, such as when a patient expresses suicidal ideation or is at immediate risk of self-harm [28]. Establishing clear protocols and local support networks are crucial to ensure patient safety in these situations.

Licensing and reimbursement issues can also pose barriers to telepsychiatry's widespread adoption. Providers need to be licensed in the state where the patient resides, which can complicate the delivery of cross-state care [29]. Moreover, although insurance coverage for telepsychiatry has improved, especially since the COVID-19 pandemic, there are still inconsistencies in reimbursement policies, with some insurers offering limited coverage compared to traditional in-person care.

In summary, telepsychiatry offers numerous benefits, including increased accessibility, continuity of care, patient comfort, and cost-effectiveness. However, it also presents challenges related to privacy, technology, the limitations of remote assessments, emergency management, licensing, and reimbursement. As telepsychiatry evolves, addressing these pitfalls will be essential to maximize its potential in mental health care delivery.

Physician to Physician Consults

Physician-to-physician virtual consultation or eConsults facilitate communication and collaboration between healthcare providers across various locations using telecommunication technologies. E-Consults allow primary care physicians (PCPs) to consult with specialists remotely, enabling more efficient, timely, and comprehensive patient care [30]. By leveraging secure messaging, video conferencing, and electronic health records (EHR) integration, eConsults bridge the gap between general practitioners and specialists, particularly benefiting healthcare systems in rural or underserved areas where access to specialty care can be limited.

One of the primary benefits of physician-to-physician virtual consultations is the ability to obtain expert input without requiring patients to make in-person specialist appointments. In many traditional healthcare settings, patients often face long wait times to see a specialist, which can delay diagnosis and treatment. eConsults can expedite this process by allowing PCPs to send relevant patient information, test results, and medical images to a specialist for review. The specialist can then provide guidance on the next steps, such as suggesting additional tests, recommending treatment adjustments, or advising whether an in-person specialist visit is necessary. This streamlined approach saves time and reduces healthcare costs by avoiding unnecessary referrals and procedures [31].

These programs also facilitate knowledge transfer and capacity building among primary care providers. By consulting with specialists through virtual platforms, PCPs can enhance their understanding of complex medical conditions and gain insights into managing a broader range of health issues within their scope of practice [32]. This collaborative model supports a more integrated approach to healthcare, improving the continuity and quality of patient care. Furthermore, it helps specialists manage their workload more effectively, allowing them to prioritize patients who genuinely need in-person evaluations.

Examples

Physician-to-physician consultation has been transformative for the healthcare system, especially within some specialized fields requiring rapid response and expert input. Key examples—such as telestroke [33] and telepediatrics [34]—demonstrate the profound impact of remote consultation capabilities on patient outcomes. These models leverage real-time video conferencing, data sharing, and remote diagnostics to provide timely access to specialists, even in regions lacking specific medical expertise. In cases of acute stroke, telestroke services allow neurologists to assess patients remotely, interpret imaging scans, and guide local physicians on optimal treatment strategies, including the use of time-sensitive interventions like thrombolytics [35]. This immediacy is crucial, as rapid treatment significantly improves outcomes in stroke patients, and without telestroke, many rural hospitals would be unable to offer this level of care.

Similarly, telepediatrics extend critical specialist support to pediatricians in underserved areas. Pediatric consultations often involve complex cases that benefit from specialist input, particularly in emergencies or when managing chronic conditions [36]. Through telepediatrics, pediatricians in remote hospitals can consult with subspecialists, access guidance on diagnostic protocols, and discuss treatment plans, ultimately enhancing the quality of pediatric care.

Other use cases of telemedicine support, like telecardiology and tele-rapid response, demonstrate the flexibility and adaptability of technology solutions to increase access to the right care at the right time. Cardiologists or emergency physicians can remotely review electrocardiograms and dramatically reduce time to life-saving interventions [37]. Tele-rapid response teams further highlight the agility of telemedicine to enable swift multidisciplinary collaboration during medical emergencies [38].

Challenges and Barriers

Despite the benefits, physician-to-physician consultation programs face several challenges. Privacy and security are significant concerns when providers transmit sensitive patient information electronically [39]. These programs must comply with regulations like the Health Insurance Portability and Accountability Act (HIPAA) to ensure the confidentiality and security of patient data. Additionally, disparities in technology access and proficiency among healthcare providers can impact the effectiveness of these virtual consultations [40]. Some providers may lack the necessary infrastructure or training to use telehealth platforms efficiently, limiting the adoption and success of such programs.

There are also reimbursement and regulatory hurdles to consider. In many regions, reimbursement policies for virtual physician-to-physician consultations are not as well-defined or consistent as those for traditional in-person visits [41, 42]. This inconsistency can create uncertainty around billing and payment for the services rendered, potentially limiting the willingness of specialists to participate in these programs. Nevertheless, as healthcare systems continue to recognize the value of virtual health programs in improving patient outcomes and care delivery efficiency, physician-to-physician consultation programs are likely to become a more integral component of healthcare.

Disaster Telemedicine

Disasters, whether natural, like a flood or a pandemic, or human-caused, like a terror attack or war, often cause resource-limited healthcare scenarios wherein local resource availability of staff, space, and "stuff" become overwhelmed. The most difficult of these resource limitations to overcome is access to knowledgeable, skilled, and experienced clinicians needed to manage patients with chronic medical conditions and casualties produced by the disaster [43]. This was acutely apparent during the COVID-19 pandemic for critical care trained clinicians. An alternative is delivering expertise with telemedicine [44].

While this solution is helpful, it has challenges related to communications networks, power, connected mobile or other hardware devices, and, most importantly, digital fluency [45]. Telemedicine may expose similar access problems to regular healthcare for underserved, socioeconomically disadvantaged, and rural demographics [46]. Nevertheless, commercial, hospital-affiliated, government and military investigators have all used telemedicine to support all phases of disaster medical response [47, 48].

Disaster Telemedicine (DTM, or disaster eHealth [DEH]) enables remote experts to expand the scope of practice for local caregivers by using technology to provide real-time, team-based care [49]. During the COVID-19 pandemic, multiple academic, commercial, and government entities supported small and large hospitals by providing expertise to the point of need [50, 51]. It has been used to augment physical healthcare delivery systems and increase access to care by facilitating triage, remote monitoring, chronic disease management, access to specialty care, mental healthcare, and prescription management. The key to the successful use of DTM is a population familiar with the technology and infrastructure, as well as a marketing plan that informs potential patients/caregivers about the availability of the service. These solutions are generally considered "alternates" when the primary plan of going to a physical healthcare facility is unavailable due to road closures, flooding, mass casualty events that overwhelm the local system, or when the local system is closed due to damage [52].

RPM also has significant potential to improve disaster medical response systems [53]. No large-scale implementation of RPM has yet been utilized during a disaster. Still, a DH ecosystem designed to optimize patient regulation and resource allocation during a disaster medical response could significantly improve patient outcomes by matching resources to patient needs most efficiently and accurately.

Innovations in Digital Health Technologies

The Advanced Research Projects Agency—Health's Platform Accelerating Rural Access to Distributed and Integrated Medical Care (ARPA-H's PARADIGM) Program seeks to reduce health inequities in rural parts of America by creating a scalable physical platform that provides access to advanced medical services outside of a hospital setting [54]. PARADIGM brings together a collection of technologies from telemedicine and remote monitoring to miniaturization of medical devices and novel power solutions that enable advanced imaging and laboratory assessments, to AI and clinical decision support, to advances in networking, cellular, and satellite communications. By integrating these technologies into a common ecosystem based on technical data and interoperability standards and deploying them within novel care delivery models, PARADIGM intends to reduce health inequities and improve patient outcomes despite resource limitations inherent to many rural communities.

Telerobotic Surgery

Telesurgery presents an opportunity to increase the availability and capacity of surgical resources when needed to care for patients in remote or resource-limited care contexts. Technology advancements have profoundly transformed surgical care, empowering surgeons to perform complex procedures with greater precision and confidence while minimizing risks and enhancing patient recovery. Technological advancements, including high-speed internet, telepresence, robotic surgical systems, and secure data transmission and encryption, coupled with the accelerated adoption of telemedicine are transforming surgical care. Surgeons now regularly perform real-time intra-operative consultations using telemedicine solutions.

In 2001, a surgical team in New York performed the first transatlantic robotic telesurgery (RTS) procedure, successfully removing the gallbladder of a patient in France [55]. Just over two decades later, in February 2024, the U.S. sent a miniature medical robot to the International Space Station and completed the first telerobotic surgery demonstration on simulated tissue in zero gravity. The robot was remotely operated by surgeons from approximately 250 miles (400 km) below in Lincoln, Nebraska [56]. Chinese surgeons have embraced and employed RTS as a civil capability to address population needs in remote population centers. The longest RTS (round trip) from Rome to Beijing (~10,000 mi) was performed in 2023 [57]. These milestones reflect continued progress in developing this technology and have profound implications for establishing access to advanced medical care in remote areas, during disaster medical responses, or wherever surgical emergencies could happen, and the necessary surgical expertise is not locally available.

Integration with Artificial Intelligence (AI)

The integration of AI with telehealth and RPM technologies holds immense potential for improving healthcare delivery. AI can enhance the accuracy of diagnostics, predict health outcomes, and personalize treatment plans based on real-time data from RPM devices. For example, AI algorithms can analyze data from wearable devices to detect early signs of health deterioration and alert healthcare providers.

Improved Interoperability and Data Sharing

For virtual health technologies to reach their full potential, improvements in interoperability and data sharing between different healthcare systems are essential. Standardizing data formats and developing secure platforms for data exchange will facilitate better coordination of care across different providers and settings.

Regulatory and Policy Developments

As the adoption of virtual health technologies increases, regulatory and policy frameworks will continue to evolve. Governments and healthcare organizations must address issues related to data privacy, security, reimbursement, and practitioner licensing to support the widespread use of telehealth and RPM. See Chap. 12 for more details on privacy rules laws and Chap. 14 for regulatory frameworks.

Enhancing Patient Experience and Engagement

Future innovations in virtual health technologies will focus on enhancing patient experience and engagement. This includes the development of user-friendly interfaces, personalized health recommendations, and support systems to encourage patients to actively participate in their care.

Conclusion

Virtual health technologies, including telehealth and remote monitoring, have fundamentally transformed healthcare delivery, offering benefits such as improved access to care, cost savings, and enhanced patient engagement [11]. However, challenges such as technological barriers, regulatory complexities, and privacy concerns must be addressed to fully realize the potential of these technologies. As healthcare continues to evolve, the integration of AI, the expansion of hospital-at-home programs, and advancements in data interoperability will drive the future of virtual health. By addressing current challenges and embracing innovation, virtual health technologies can significantly improve healthcare outcomes and enhance the quality of life for patients worldwide.

Acknowledgements Jeremy C. Pamplin, MD, FCCM, FACP provided valuable insights, editorial advice, and original material about eConsults in emergencies and disaster telehealth. He is affiliated with the U.S. Army Telemedicine and Advanced Technology Research Center, Frederick, MD, USA and a Professor of Medicine and Military and Emergency Medicine at the Uniformed Services University of the Health Sciences, Bethesda, MD, USA.

Disclaimer "The views, opinions, and/or findings contained in this research/presentation/ publication are those of the author(s)/company and do not necessarily reflect the views of the Department of Defense and should not be construed as an official DoD/Army position, policy or decision unless so designated by other documentation. No official endorsement should be made.

References

1. Tan SY, Sumner J, Wang Y, Wenjun Yip A. A systematic review of the impacts of remote patient monitoring (RPM) interventions on safety, adherence, quality-of-life, and cost-related outcomes. NPJ Digit Med. 2024;7(1):192.
2. de Sousa Vale J, Franco AI, Oliveira CV, Araújo I, Sousa D. Hospital at home: an overview of the literature. Home Health Care Manag Pract. 2020;32(2):118–23.
3. Santosa KB, Cederna PS. Commentary on: Trends and challenges of telehealth in an academic institution: the unforeseen benefits of the COVID-19 global pandemic. Aesthet Surg J. 2021;41(1):119–21.
4. World Health Organization. WHO Guideline: recommendations on digital interventions for health system strengthening; 2020. https://www.who.int/publications/i/item/9789241550505. Accessed 19 Sept 2024.
5. Leff B, Levine DM, Siu AL. The acute hospital care at home waiver and the future of hospital at home in the US. Health Affairs, May 3, 2024.
6. Curfman A, Hackell JM, Herendeen NE, Alexander J, Marcin JP, Moskowitz WB, et al. Telehealth: opportunities to improve access, quality, and cost in pediatric care. Pediatrics. 2022;149(3):e2021056035.
7. American Medical Association. Telehealth implementation playbook; 2020. https://www.ama-assn.org/system/files/2020-04/ama-telehealth-playbook.pdf. Accessed 19 Sept 2024.
8. Short Apellaniz J, Álvaro de la Parra JA, Gomez-Meana A, Carabias L, Cordoba R, Arcos J, Blanco Á, et al. Leveraging telemedicine to reduce ED overcrowding: The Quirónsalud Virtual Urgent Care Program. NEJM Catal Innov Care Deliv. 2023;4(8):CAT-22.
9. Ong MK, Romano PS, Edgington S, Aronow HU, Auerbach AD, Black JT, et al. Effectiveness of remote patient monitoring after discharge of hospitalized patients with heart failure: the better effectiveness after transition–heart failure (BEAT-HF) randomized clinical trial. JAMA Intern Med. 2016;176(3):310–8.
10. Klersy C, Boriani G, De Silvestri A, Mairesse GH, Braunschweig F, Scotti V, et al. Effect of telemonitoring of cardiac implantable electronic devices on healthcare utilization: a meta-analysis of randomized controlled trials in patients with heart failure. Eur J Heart Fail. 2016;18(2):195–204.
11. Koehler F, Koehler K, Deckwart O, Prescher S, Wegscheider K, Kirwan BA, et al. Efficacy of telemedical interventional management in patients with heart failure (TIM-HF2): a randomised, controlled, parallel-group, unmasked trial. Lancet. 2018;392(10152):1047–57.
12. Al-Naher A, Downing J, Scott KA, Pirmohamed M. Factors affecting patient and physician engagement in remote health care for heart failure: systematic review. JMIR Cardiol. 2022;6(1):e33366.

13. Ramachandran M, Brinton C, Wiljer D, Upshur R, Gray C. The impact of eHealth on relationships and trust in primary care: a review of reviews. BMC Prim Care. 2023;24(1). https://doi.org/10.1186/s12875-023-02176-5.
14. Silva E, Breslau J, Barr RM, Liebscher LA, Bohl M, Hoffman T, et al. ACR white paper on teleradiology practice: a report from the Task Force on Teleradiology Practice. J Am Coll Radiol. 2013;10(8):575–85.
15. Hanna TN, Scott D, Steenburg SD, Pyatt RS Jr, Duszak R Jr, Friedberg EB. Emerging challenges and opportunities in the evolution of teleradiology. Am J Roentgenol. 2020;215(6):1411–8.
16. White P. Privacy and security issues in teleradiology. Semin Ultrasound CT MR. 2004;25(5):391–5.
17. Satyanarayanan M, et al. Security requirements for teleradiology systems. IEEE Trans Inf Technol Biomed. 2006;10(1):75–84.
18. Krupinski EA. Quality control in teleradiology. J Am Coll Radiol. 2014;11(12):1159–64.
19. Armstrong AW, Wu J. Teledermatology: a comprehensive overview. J Am Acad Dermatol. 2012;67(5):933–48.
20. Datta SK, Warshaw EM. Effectiveness of teledermatology in providing dermatologic care to underserved populations. Telemed e-Health. 2010;16(4):354–60.
21. Trettel A, Eissing L, Augustin M. Patient and provider satisfaction with teledermatology: a systematic review and Meta-analysis. JAMA Dermatol. 2018;154(6):748–56.
22. Esteva A, Kuprel B, Thrun S. Artificial intelligence in dermatology: current applications and future prospects. Nature. 2017;542(7639):115–8.
23. Villani A, et al. Teledermatology during the COVID-19 pandemic: experience of an academic center. Clin Exp Dermatol. 2020;45(7):891–4.
24. Shore JH, Stec B, Tomblin S, Coustasse A. Telepsychiatry in the 21st century: transforming healthcare delivery. Psychiatr Clin N Am. 2018;41(4):533–46.
25. Hubley S, Lynch SB, Schneck C, et al. Patient satisfaction with telepsychiatry services. Can J Psychiatr. 2016;61(10):688–92.
26. Yellowlees P, et al. Telepsychiatry: enhancing mental health care through remote technology. World Psychiatry. 2017;16(1):87–8.
27. Perakovic M, et al. Security and privacy challenges in telemedicine and eHealth: a survey. J Health Inf Res. 2018;4(4):127–34.
28. Gros DF, et al. The challenges of telepsychiatry for rural populations. J Rural Ment Health. 2013;37(2):64–72.
29. O'Reilly R, et al. Telepsychiatry for the management of mental health in primary care: a systematic review. Can J Psychiatr. 2007;52(9):607–16.
30. Thomas JF, et al. Licensure and reimbursement barriers to telemedicine implementation in child psychiatry. J Am Acad Child Adolesc Psychiatry. 2020;59(5):539–47.
31. Thompson MA, Fuhlbrigge AL, Pearson DW, Saxon DR, Oberst-Walsh LA, Thomas JF. Building eConsult (Electronic Consults) capability at an academic medical center to improve efficiencies in delivering specialty care. J Prim Care Community Health. 2021;12:21501327211005303.
32. Vimalananda VG, et al. The impact of electronic consultation on efficiency and cost in specialty care delivery. Telemed e-Health. 2015;21(12):1038–46.
33. Lazarus G, Permana AP, Nugroho SW, Audrey J, Wijaya DN, Widyahening IS. Telestroke strategies to enhance acute stroke management in rural settings: a systematic review and meta-analysis. Brain Behav. 2020;10(10):e01787.
34. Nadar M, Jouvet P, Tucci M, Toledano B, Sicotte C. Impact of synchronous telemedicine models on clinical outcomes in pediatric acute care settings: a systematic review. Pediatr Crit Care Med. 2018;19(12):e662–71.
35. Mohamed A, Elsherif S, Legere B, Fatima N, Shuaib A, Saqqur M. Is telestroke more effective than conventional treatment for acute ischemic stroke? A systematic review and meta-analysis of patient outcomes and thrombolysis rates. Int J Stroke. 2024;19(3):280–92.
36. Shah AC, Badawy SM. Telemedicine in pediatrics: systematic review of randomized controlled trials. JMIR Pediatr Parent. 2021;4(1):e22696.

37. Brunetti ND, De Gennaro L, Correale M, Santoro F, Caldarola P, Gaglione A, Di Biase M. Prehospital electrocardiogram triage with telemedicine near halves time to treatment in STEMI: a meta-analysis and meta-regression analysis of non-randomized studies. Int J Cardiol. 2017;232:5–11.
38. Pappas PA, Tirelli L, Shaffer J, Gettings S. Projecting critical care beyond the ICU: an analysis of tele-ICU support for rapid response teams. Telemed e-Health. 2016;22(6):529–33.
39. Liddy C, Afkham A, Drosinis P, Joschko J, Keely E. Impact of and satisfaction with a new eConsult service: a mixed methods study of primary care providers. J Am Board Fam Med. 2015;28(3):394–403.
40. McMahon GT, Mermelstein AM. Implementing eConsult systems: considerations for privacy and security. J Ambul Care Manage. 2013;36(2):122–8.
41. Liddy C, et al. Barriers and facilitators to using eConsult services: perspectives of primary care providers and specialists. J Telemed Telecare. 2016;22(6):361–6.
42. Anderson D, Aoki N. Reimbursement models for eConsult services: opportunities and challenges. Am J Manag Care. 2016;22(10):747–52.
43. The Society of Critical Care Medicine. Fundamentals of critical care support: crisis management. Chapter 3. In: Augmenting critical care capacity during a disaster; 2022. Chicago. p. 1–10.
44. Barbash IJ, Sackrowitz RE, Gajic O, Dempsey TM, Bell S, Millerman K, et al. Rapidly deploying critical care telemedicine across states and health systems during the Covid-19 pandemic. NEJM Catal Innov Care Deliv. 2020;1(4). https://doi.org/10.1056/CAT.20.0301.
45. Vogels EA. Digital gap between rural and non rural America persists. Pew Research Center Fact Tank. 2019. https://www.pewresearch.org/fact-tank/2019/05/31/digital-gap-between-rural-and-nonrural-america-per-sists/. Accessed 24 Oct 2024.
46. Park JH, Lee MJ, Tsai MH, Shih HJ, Chang J. Rural, regional, racial disparities in telemedicine use during the COVID-19 pandemic among US adults: 2021 National Health Interview Survey (NHIS). Patient Prefer Adherence. 2023; p. 3477–87.
47. Litvak M, Miller K, Boyle T, et al. Telemedicine use in disasters: a scoping review. Disaster Med Public Health Prep. 2022;16(2):791–800.
48. Salehinejad S, Jannati N, Ershad Sarabi R, Bahaadinbeigy K. Use of telemedicine and e-health in disasters: a systematic review. J Emerg Pract Trauma. 2021;7(1):56–62.
49. Madanian S, Norris T, Parry D. Disaster eHealth: scoping review. J Med Internet Res. 2020;22(10):e18310.
50. Wosik J, Fudim M, Cameron B, Gellad ZF, Cho A, Phinney D, et al. Telehealth transformation: COVID-19 and the rise of virtual care. J Am Med Inform Assoc. 2020;27(6):957–62.
51. Boyle TP, Mehra A, Smith NJ, Subramanian S, Leeber J, McMahon M, et al. The first statewide implementation of a regional disaster teleconsultation system to expand critical care surge capacity: a case study in Vermont. Telemed e-Health. 2024;30(5):1495–8.
52. American College of Emergency Physicians. Disaster telehealth policy statement. Approved January 2024. https://www.acep.org/patient-care/policy-statements/disaster-telehealth. Accessed 31 Oct 2024.
53. Pamplin JC, Gray B, Quinn MT, Little JR, Colombo CJ, Subramanian S, Governance Stakeholder Working Group and National Emergency Tele-Critical Care Network Team Participants, et al. National emergency tele-critical care in a pandemic: barriers and solutions. Crit Care Explor. 2024;6(5):e1091.
54. The Advanced Research Projects Agency for Health Platform Accelerating Rural Access to Distributed and Integrated Medical Care (ARPA-H PARADIGM) Program at https://arpa-h.gov/research-and-funding/programs/paradigm. Accessed 22 Oct 2024.
55. Gottlieb S. Surgeons perform transatlantic operation using fibreoptics. BMJ. 2001;323(7315):713.
56. Kim J. A tiny robot on the space station will simulate remote-controlled surgery up there. NPR News. Published February 12, 2024. https://www.npr.org. Accessed 1 Nov 2024.
57. Copestake J. Chinese team perform world-first robotic surgery from Rome in Beijing. CGTN. Published June 12, 2024. https://newseu.cgtn.com/news/2024-06-12/Chinese-team-perform-world-first-robotic-surgery-from-Rome-in-Beijing-1um4yx45Ixq/p.html. Accessed 1 Nov 2024.

Chapter 3
Health Informatics

Thomas J. Cantilina

Introduction

Health informatics (HI) is an interdisciplinary field that applies the use of information technology (IT) to improve healthcare delivery and patient outcomes [1]. The practitioners in the field are experts in the integration of people, process, and technology. In today's healthcare arena the practice of medicine has become extraordinarily complex and specialized for all roles, not just for physicians. Understanding how to ensure technology is an enabler rather than an obstacle is the core mission of health informatics. While there are many ways to approach technology, an easy to remember way is to group technologies as the three "D's: Desktop (software), Devices (hardware from ultrasounds to mobile computers), and Data (the output or storage of electrons created by either the desktop or device).

This chapter describes the multifaceted field of health informatics, beginning with an examination of its definition and scope. Health Informatics encompasses the application of IT and information management principles to healthcare delivery, evolving from the digitization of medical records to sophisticated systems that support clinical decision-making and population health management.

The Field of Health Informatics

Health informatics involves a wide range of activities, from the collection, organization, and storage of health data to the development of clinical decision support tools and the implementation of electronic health records (EHRs) [2]. Health informatics

T. J. Cantilina (✉)
Formerly Department of Defense, Defense Health Agency, Falls Church, VA, USA
e-mail: thomas.cantilina@doctomcan.net

T. Adirim (ed.), *Digital Health, AI and Generative AI in Healthcare*,
https://doi.org/10.1007/978-3-031-83526-1_3

professionals work to bridge the gap between healthcare providers, patients, and technology, ensuring that health information is accurate, accessible, and actionable [3]. While the EHR is a cornerstone of this work, it is just the tip of the iceberg. The field's early beginnings emerged in the 1950s when hospitals started using computers to automate administrative tasks. Pioneers during this era began to utilize this data to explore medical decision support systems. By the 1970s the term "medical informatics" was coined, with the focus expanding to EHRs, hospital information systems, and the initial development of standards for exchanging health information (i.e., Health Level-7, Digital Imaging and Communications in Medicine) [4].

The internet further revolutionized health informatics, enabling telemedicine, online resources, and data-driven research. EHRs became more sophisticated, and health information exchange gained momentum with the passage of the Health Information Technology for Economic and Clinical Health Act (HITECH) in 2009 [5]. This landmark legislation significantly changed the healthcare playing field by accelerating the adoption of Electronic Health Records (EHRs) in the United States. Enacted in 2009 as part of the American Recovery and Reinvestment Act, HITECH aimed to promote the widespread use of health information technology with the intention to improve the quality, safety, and efficiency of healthcare delivery. It accomplished this acceleration in five key ways:

1. Provided financial Incentives: HITECH provided Medicare and Medicaid reimbursements to healthcare providers, primarily hospitals and physicians, who demonstrated "meaningful use" of certified EHR technology, making EHR adoption financially attractive.
2. Established meaningful use criteria: HITECH established a set of "meaningful use" criteria that outlined specific objectives for EHR use, such as electronic prescribing, clinical decision support, and health information exchange. These criteria encouraged healthcare providers to adopt EHRs and utilize them in ways that could improve patient care.
3. Improved EHR Certification: HITECH led to the development of more rigorous certification standards for EHR technology. These standards ensured that EHR systems met specific requirements for functionality, interoperability, and security, making them more reliable and trustworthy for healthcare providers.
4. Directed penalties for non-compliance: HITECH also introduced penalties for healthcare providers who failed to adopt and meaningfully use EHR technology. These penalties, in the form of reduced Medicare and Medicaid reimbursements, created a sense of urgency for EHR adoption.
5. Promoted improved health information exchange: HITECH promoted the development of health information exchange (HIE) networks, which facilitated the secure sharing of patient health information between healthcare providers and organizations. This was meant to improve care coordination and reduce unnecessary duplication of services.

EHR usage soared from 3.2% prior to the passage of HITECH to 86% of office-based physicians and 96% of non-federal acute care hospitals adopting EHRs by 2017 [6]. While HITECH was instrumental in driving EHR adoption, it also faced some criticisms, such as concerns about the usability of EHR systems and the potential for information overload for healthcare providers. These concerns created the landscape for the development of health informatics as a career field. Its overall impact on accelerating EHR adoption and improving healthcare delivery is widely recognized despite early critics.

Information technology continues its exponential growth and innovation and therefore health informaticists need to understand subjects such as natural language processing (NLP), big data, machine learning, cloud computing, mobile devices, cybersecurity, health information exchange, "bots", ambient listening, robotics, interfaces, and interoperability to leverage health IT outputs for greater effectiveness and efficiency of healthcare. Ultimately, if something uses an electron to store or move information, it is in the realm of informatics, and it becomes health informatics when these electrons are used to improve patient outcomes as well as patient or provider experience.

Who Works in Health Informatics?

The foundation of an effective health informaticist is an experienced healthcare professional: doctors, nurses, pharmacists, and other clinicians who understand first-hand how healthcare is delivered. Additionally, a clinical background is critical to translate the needs of the clinician to the technology developers and in turn are the trusted sources to communicate to clinical peers how the technology works. While the skills of an informaticist benefit healthcare at any level of care, from the ambulatory physician's office to the multi-facility integrated hospital and referral system, the dedicated health informaticist is more likely to work in hospitals and healthcare systems [7, 8]. The bigger the system, the bigger the need for an informaticist's expertise. Departments of health informatics in hospital systems usually contain one or many of the following roles:

- Health Informatics Specialists: These professionals have a strong foundation in both healthcare and IT. They may work as data analysts, system administrators, or project managers, contributing to the design, implementation, and maintenance of health information systems.
- Clinical Informaticists: These are healthcare professionals (e.g., physicians, nurses, pharmacists) with additional training in informatics. They work at the intersection of clinical practice and technology, utilizing their expertise to improve patient care using IT.
- Health Information Managers (HIM): HIM professionals are responsible for the overall management of health information, ensuring its quality, integrity, and security. They may work in hospitals, clinics, or other healthcare settings.
- Data Scientists: With the increasing volume and complexity of health data, data scientists play a crucial role in analyzing and interpreting this information to uncover insights that can inform clinical decision-making and improve population

health. These members of the informatics team have expertise in computer science and data analytics.

Certifications and Education

While there are no universally mandatory certifications for all health informatics roles, several certifications can enhance professional credibility and demonstrate expertise. Some of the most recognized certifications include:

- Registered Health Information Administrator (RHIA): Offered by the American Health Information Management Association (AHIMA), this certification is designed for HIM professionals.
- Certified Health Data Analyst (CHDA): Also offered by AHIMA, this certification focuses on data analysis skills for health informatics professionals.
- Certified Professional in Healthcare Information and Management Systems (CPHIMS): Offered by the Healthcare Information and Management Systems Society (HIMSS), this certification is broader in scope and covers various aspects of health informatics.

The choice of certification often depends on the specific career path and interests of the individual. Some roles may require or strongly prefer candidates with specific certifications.

Since 2013 board certified physicians in a multitude of specialties can now get a secondary board certification in clinical informatics through the American Board of Preventive Medicine (ABPM). This requires completing an approved fellowship in health informatics at an accredited institution. The field is constantly evolving, and new roles and certifications are emerging.

Scope of Practice

Health informatics professionals play a pivotal role in the development of health IT solutions and software, leveraging their expertise in both healthcare and technology to create innovative tools that improve patient care, streamline workflows, and enhance healthcare delivery [9]. Their scope of practice in this domain is extensive and multifaceted, encompassing the following key areas:

- *Needs Assessment and Requirement Analysis*: Health informatics professionals collaborate with healthcare providers, administrators, and other stakeholders to identify pain points, challenges, and unmet needs in the healthcare system. They conduct thorough needs assessments and requirement analysis to determine the specific functionalities and features that a health IT solution should possess to address these issues effectively.

- *System Design and Development*: Health informaticists contribute to the design and development of health IT solutions, ensuring that they align with clinical workflows, regulatory requirements, and industry best practices. They participate in the selection of appropriate technologies, data models, and user interfaces, ensuring that the final products are user-friendly, efficient, and scalable.
- *Implementation and Integration*: Health informatics professionals oversee the implementation and integration of health IT solutions into existing healthcare systems. They work closely with IT teams to ensure seamless data exchange, interoperability, and compatibility with other software applications. They also provide training and support to end-users, ensuring smooth adoption and utilization of the new technology.
- *Testing and Quality Assurance*: Health informaticists play a critical role in the processes that ensure the health IT solution functions as intended and meets all safety and performance standards. They conduct rigorous testing to identify and rectify any bugs, errors, or inconsistencies, rendering the final product reliable, accurate, and secure.
- *Data Analytics and Evaluation*: Health informatics professionals utilize their data analytics skills to evaluate the effectiveness and impact of health IT solutions. They collect and analyze data on user adoption, system performance, and patient outcomes to identify areas for improvement and optimize the functionality of the solution. They also conduct post-implementation evaluations to assess the technology's long-term benefits and return on investment.
- *Maintenance and Support*: Health informaticists provide ongoing maintenance and support for health IT solutions, ensuring their continued functionality and relevance in the ever-evolving healthcare landscape. They address any technical issues; update software as needed and provide training and guidance to users.

AI is transforming the field of health informatics by including requirements for skills in machine learning, management and training of datasets and implementation within and in addition to EHRs to ensure AI applications are safely and responsibly used by medical personnel. By actively engaging in these diverse aspects of health IT solution development, health informatics professionals contribute to the advancement of healthcare technology, ultimately improving patient care, reducing healthcare costs, and enhancing the overall efficiency and effectiveness of the healthcare system.

HI Role within Healthcare Institutions

Health informatics professionals significantly impact healthcare operations, optimizing processes, enhancing efficiency, and improving patient care delivery. Their scope of practice in this domain is vast and encompasses various critical areas:

- *Process Improvement and Optimization*: Health informaticists analyze existing healthcare workflows and identify bottlenecks, inefficiencies, and areas for improvement. They leverage their knowledge of healthcare operations and information systems to design and implement solutions that streamline processes, reduce redundancies, and enhance overall productivity.

- *Electronic Health Record (EHR) Implementation and Optimization*: Health informatics professionals play a central role in the implementation and optimization of EHR systems. They ensure that the EHR is configured to meet the specific needs of the organization, integrates with other health IT systems, and complies with regulatory requirements. They also train staff on the use of the EHR and provide ongoing support to maximize its benefits.
- *Data Management and Analytics*: Health informaticists are responsible for managing and analyzing vast amounts of healthcare data generated by various sources, including EHRs, medical devices, and clinical trials. They use their expertise in data analytics to derive meaningful insights that inform clinical decision-making, improve patient outcomes, and enhance operational efficiency.
- *Performance Measurement and Reporting*: Health informatics professionals develop and implement performance measurement systems to track key healthcare metrics, such as patient satisfaction, readmission rates, and length of stay. They generate reports that provide actionable insights to healthcare leaders, enabling them to make data-driven decisions to improve quality of care and operational efficiency.
- *Resource Management and Allocation*: Health informaticists utilize data analytics to optimize resource allocation, ensuring that staff, equipment, and supplies are deployed efficiently to meet patient demand. They develop scheduling algorithms, forecast patient volumes, and identify opportunities for cost savings, ultimately enhancing the financial sustainability of healthcare organizations.
- *Risk Management and Compliance*: Health informatics professionals play a crucial role in risk management and compliance, ensuring that healthcare organizations adhere to regulatory requirements and industry standards. They develop and implement policies and procedures to protect patient privacy, ensure data security, and mitigate the risk of medical errors.
- *Health Information Exchange (HIE)*: Health informaticists facilitate the secure exchange of health information between different healthcare providers and organizations, enabling seamless care coordination and improving patient outcomes. They participate in the development and implementation of HIE networks, ensuring that data is transmitted securely and efficiently.

In many healthcare organizations, health informaticists have ascended to leadership roles within the C-suite, reflecting the growing importance of data-driven decision-making and the strategic value of health information. This elevated position allows them to directly influence organizational strategy, advocate for technology investments, and drive innovation in healthcare delivery.

The specific job titles for health informaticists in the C-suite can vary depending on the size and structure of the organization. Some common titles include:

- *Chief Health Informatics Officer (CHIO)*: This is a senior executive position responsible for overseeing the organization's health informatics strategy,

ensuring alignment with overall business goals, and promoting the effective use of HIT to improve patient care and operational efficiency.
- *Chief Medical Information Officer (CMIO)*: This is a position typically held by a physician with expertise in informatics. The CMIO focuses on the clinical applications of HIT, ensuring that technology solutions are designed to meet the needs of clinicians and enhance patient care.
- *Chief Nursing Information Officer (CNIO)*: This role is similar to the CMIO but focuses on the nursing perspective, ensuring that HIT supports nursing workflows, improves patient safety, and enhances the nursing profession.
- *Chief Information Officer (CIO) (*with a Health Informatics Focus): In some organizations, the CIO may have a strong background in health informatics and oversee both general IT functions and the specific needs of healthcare technology.

Additionally, in recent years, a new senior health care leader position has emerged, the Chief AI Officer (CAIO). The CAIO has similar skills as CMIO and CHIO, but in addition has skills in machine learning, training of data, and piloting of AI applications and is responsible for the organization's AI strategy. Regardless of the specific title, health informaticists in the C-suite typically have a broad range of responsibilities, including:

- Developing and implementing a comprehensive health informatics strategy that aligns with the organization's mission, vision, and strategic goals.
- Advocating for investments in HIT and ensuring that technology solutions are implemented effectively and integrated seamlessly into existing workflows.
- Leading the development and implementation of data governance policies and procedures to ensure the quality, integrity, and security of health information.
- Collaborating with clinical and administrative leaders to identify opportunities for improvement and leverage HIT to enhance patient care, streamline operations, and reduce costs.
- Promoting a culture of data-driven decision-making throughout the organization by providing training, education, and support to staff at all levels.
- Staying abreast of emerging trends and technologies in health informatics and evaluating their potential impact on the organization.

Health informaticists employ a variety of methods to find and utilize data to enhance patient care, leveraging both internal and external sources to gain valuable insights. They analyze this data to identify patterns, trends, and areas for improvement, ultimately leading to better clinical decision-making and enhanced patient outcomes.

Datasets used by health informaticists for data analysis and to support development of AI applications include:

Electronic Health Records: EHRs serve as a primary source of patient data for health informaticists. They contain a wealth of information, including medical history, diagnoses, treatments, medications, allergies, and laboratory results. Health informaticists can query EHRs to identify specific patient populations, track disease trends, and assess treatment outcomes. For example, a health informaticist might analyze EHR data to identify patients with a particular chronic condition, such as diabetes.

They can then track these patients' progress over time, assess the effectiveness of different treatment plans, and identify potential interventions to improve outcomes.

Clinical Data Registries: Clinical data registries are databases that collect standardized data on specific diseases or conditions, providing valuable information on disease prevalence, treatment patterns, and long-term outcomes. Health informaticists can use registry data to compare their institution's performance to national benchmarks, identify areas for improvement, and develop targeted interventions. For example, a health informaticist working in a cancer center might utilize a national cancer registry to compare their institution's survival rates for a specific type of cancer to national averages. If their rates are lower, they can investigate potential reasons and implement changes to improve patient care.

Administrative and Claims Data: Administrative and claims data include information on patient demographics, insurance coverage, billing codes, and hospital utilization. Health informaticists can analyze this data to identify high-risk patient populations, track healthcare costs, and assess the financial impact of different interventions. For example, a health informaticist might analyze claims data to identify patients who are frequently hospitalized for a particular condition. They can then develop targeted interventions to reduce hospitalizations and improve care coordination for these patients.

Patient-Generated Health Data (PGHD): PGHD includes data collected from patients themselves, such as through wearable devices, mobile apps, or online surveys. This data can provide valuable insights into patients' daily lives, health behaviors, and experiences with their care. Health informaticists can use PGHD to personalize care plans, monitor patient progress, and engage patients in their own health management. For example, a health informaticist might use data from a patient's wearable device to track their physical activity levels and sleep patterns. This information can be used to identify potential health risks and develop personalized interventions to improve the patient's overall health.

Public Health Data: This includes data collected by government agencies and other organizations on population health trends, disease outbreaks, and environmental factors that can affect health. Health informaticists can use public health data to identify emerging health threats, track the spread of infectious diseases, and assess the impact of public health interventions.

For example, a health informaticist working in a public health department might analyze data on influenza vaccination rates to identify populations with low vaccination coverage and develop targeted outreach programs to increase vaccination rates.

Role within Public Health

Health informatics crosses into the realm of public health when the focus moves from efficiency and effectiveness to surveillance and population impact [10]. Due to the collection, storage, integration (interoperability), and analysis of big data, health informatics is making huge strides in public health such as:

- *Disease Surveillance and Outbreak Detection*: Health informatics systems enable the collection and analysis of health data from various sources, such as electronic health records, disease registries, and laboratory reports. This information helps identify disease trends, detect outbreaks early, and monitor the spread of infectious diseases.
- *Public Health Surveillance*: Health informatics tools facilitate the collection and analysis of data on health behaviors, risk factors, and environmental exposures. This information helps identify populations at risk, assess the effectiveness of public health interventions, and guide the allocation of resources.
- *Health Promotion and Disease Prevention*: Health informatics supports the development and implementation of health promotion and disease prevention programs. By analyzing health data, public health officials can identify target populations, tailor interventions, and evaluate the impact of programs.
- *Healthcare Quality Improvement*: Health informatics plays a vital role in measuring and improving the quality of healthcare services. By analyzing healthcare data, public health officials can identify areas for improvement, implement quality improvement initiatives, and monitor progress.
- *Public Health Decision-Making*: Health informatics provides evidence-based information to support public health decision-making. By analyzing health data, public health officials can assess the impact of policies and programs, identify emerging health threats, and allocate resources effectively.
- *Health Equity*: Health informatics can help identify and address health disparities among different populations. By analyzing health data by race, ethnicity, socioeconomic status, and other factors, public health officials can identify populations with disproportionate disease burdens and tailor interventions to address their specific needs.

See Chap. 9 for more details on AI use in public health.

The Informaticist's Role in Data Management

Without big data (and massive computing power) there is no AI. Leveraging data for more than just the storage of records is the impetus for and the foundation of health informatics. Just as the development of the computer enabled the capture of life as a snapshot stored as electrons, so collecting, storing, moving, and analyzing data led to the emerging of the field of informatics in the 1960s. In the subsequent decades of the 1990s and 2000s, the focus shifted to designing better ways to *collect* data through manual entry during workflow or automation through devices. This was soon followed by improved *storage* capacity with huge server farms we now call "the cloud" which brought us into the current era of big data. Big data references the three V's:

- Volume—the amount of data collected (i.e., in the terabyte and exabyte range from sensors, consolidation, images, etc.)

- Velocity—the rate at which data is acquired (i.e., how fast data is generated and collected now in milliseconds rather than weeks or days)
- Variety—the format the data is stored as (i.e., text, images, videos, structured, unstructured, vector maps, etc.)

A solid understanding of data standards and how to leverage them to promote interoperability is then key for the *movement* of data. The establishment of definable attributes of data to facilitate integration of data from multiple sources, and storage methodologies such as structured data in relational databases (e.g., Excel files, SQL databases) and unstructured data (e.g., text files, documents, images, and videos) is critical to move the data from place to place. Lastly, the more tangible work is done through the *analysis* of the data. It must be re-emphasized that without the acquisition, storage, and ability to move data, any analysis would be impossible. Likewise, without an understanding of how analytics are performed, finding useful information from the data is impossible [11].

In this vein, the date lifecycle is this: the science of taking 0s and 1s (binary data), turning them into human-readable data, which then can be analyzed to better understand health care. This process, in essence, can be summarized as the collected data representing information (i.e. the health record, population statistics), which improves knowledge (i.e. the course of disease over time or the impact of disease across a population), and which eventually gives us wisdom (i.e. the insight needed to change the course of disease). Put into more practical terms, data goes from transactional (individual records) to automation (i.e., using a previous entered address to make a mailing label or height and weight to display BMI) followed by lists (data across multiple records) giving us the *information* we need for analysis. The process of turning this *information* into *knowledge*, starts with descriptive statistics (i.e., incidence of a disease within a certain population) that can become predictive statistics giving us the probability or better the degree of certainty what will happen. This in turn brings us to prescriptive statistics which is the *wisdom* to know what to do with the knowledge we have gained through descriptive and predictive statistics.

This progressive use of data with less and less human intervention has led us to where we are today in artificial intelligence. Health informaticists understand how a state or action became an electron, which is how it was collected or turned into data, the format in which it was originally stored, and the provenance or how it got to where it is being used for integration and analysis. It is for just these reasons that the role of health informaticists has become critical in leading teams of software engineers and data scientists to build systems that are accurate reflections of reality and thus trustworthy. While in some ways the field of health informatics has returned to its roots in data, in current practice, the informaticists role has matured to become a true team integrator. This evolution is needed to ensure the ethical use of artificial intelligence in medicine creating experts in both good medicine and in the latest technologies to lead this disruptive innovation.

Conclusion

Health informatics is a dynamic field that bridges the gap between healthcare and technology. Professionals in this field utilize their expertise in both domains to improve patient care, streamline operations, and enhance healthcare delivery.

Key roles and responsibilities of health informatics professionals include development of health IT solutions including AI tools, optimization of healthcare operations, leadership in healthcare institutions and data management and analysis for improved patient care. While not always mandatory, certifications such as the Registered Health Information Administrator (RHIA), Certified Health Data Analyst (CHDA), and Certified Professional in Healthcare Information and Management Systems (CPHIMS) can enhance professional credibility and demonstrate expertise.

Overall, health informatics plays a crucial role in transforming healthcare delivery by harnessing the power of data and technology to improve patient outcomes, enhance operational efficiency, and drive innovation in the healthcare industry.

References

1. Jen MY, Mechanic OJ, Teoli D. Informatics. StatPearls [Internet]. Updated September 4, 2023. https://www.ncbi.nlm.nih.gov/books/NBK470564/. Accessed 17 June 2024.
2. All You Need to Know About Health Informatics & Health Information. DENYSYS. Published November 6, 2023. https://www.denysys.com/blog/healthcare-information-systems/. Accessed 20 July 2024.
3. Sell M. What is informatics? Regis University News Posts. Published July 26, 2022. https://www.regis.edu/news/2022/discern-learn/07/what-is-health-informatics. Accessed 17 June 2024.
4. Net Health. The History of Electronic Health Records (EHRs). Published July 20, 2023. https://www.nethealth.com/blog/the-history-of-electronic-health-records-ehrs/. Accessed 29 Sept 2024.
5. U.S. Congress. Health Information Technology for Economic and Clinical Health (HITECH) Act, H.R. 1, 111th Congress; 2009. https://www.congress.gov/bill/111th-congress/house-bill/1. Accessed 29 Sept 2024.
6. Curogram. Everything You Need to Know About the HITECH Act. Published November 9, 2022. https://blog.curogram.com/everything-you-need-to-know-about-the-hitech-act. Accessed 29 Sept 2024.
7. PublicHealthDegrees.org. Health informatics careers. Published September 10, 2023. https://www.publichealthdegrees.org/careers/health-informatics/. Accessed 29 Sept 2024.
8. All Allied Health Schools. Health informatics career paths. https://www.allalliedhealthschools.com/health-informatics/career-paths/. Accessed 29 Sept 2024.

9. Wolters Kluwer. Nursing informatics: the intersection of technology and clinical practice. Published March 27, 2018. https://www.wolterskluwer.com/en/expert-insights/nursing-informatics-the-intersection-of-technology-and-clinical-practice. Accessed 29 Sept 2024.
10. Centers for Disease Control and Prevention (CDC). Public health surveillance: preparing for the future. MMWR Morb Mortal Wkly Rep. 2012;61(Suppl 3):20–4. https://www.cdc.gov/mmwr/preview/mmwrhtml/su6103a5.htm. Accessed 29 Sept 2024.
11. Houser SH, Blabac L. Data analytics concepts for health information professionals. J AHIMA. Published October 9, 2023. https://journal.ahima.org/page/data-analytics-concepts-for-health-information-professionals. Accessed 29 Sept 2024.

Chapter 4
Artificial Intelligence Fundamentals

David Carnahan

Introduction

Artificial Intelligence (AI) has been with us for decades, but not until recently have applications for healthcare been imagined and executed. Furthermore, there has been an unprecedented surge in data generation, particularly in healthcare, where medical data alone accounts for 30% of all global data production [1] with an estimated 80% of this data as unstructured data in the form of clinical notes, medical images, videos and audio files [2]. Additionally, the administrative burden in healthcare has increased with an escalating requirement to report digital measures; most of which are due to the push by payers to change the healthcare delivery paradigm from fee for service to value-based care. All these darkening clouds portend a stormy future for clinicians unless we can use technology to mitigate these forces. So, as healthcare navigates a data-rich, information poor, administratively challenging landscape, artificial intelligence (AI) rises as a potential tool to help clinicians tap into this vast amount of information with the promise of improving patient care.

This chapter introduces clinicians to the basics of AI in healthcare, exploring its uses, purpose, and potential applications. We'll examine how advanced computing, big data processing, and sophisticated algorithms have propelled AI into the spotlight, offering new ways to analyze complex medical data, assist in diagnosis, and personalize treatment plans. However, we'll also address the challenges that come with implementing AI in healthcare, including ethical and data privacy concerns, and the need for clinical validation. As we delve into this emerging field, we'll equip you with the knowledge to understand AI's potential role in shaping the future of medicine. To build this understanding, we'll examine a framework that breaks down AI's core components, exploring how different AI systems adapt to specific

D. Carnahan (✉)
Amazon Web Services, Worldwide Public Sector, San Antonio, TX, USA

T. Adirim (ed.), *Digital Health, AI and Generative AI in Healthcare*,
https://doi.org/10.1007/978-3-031-83526-1_4

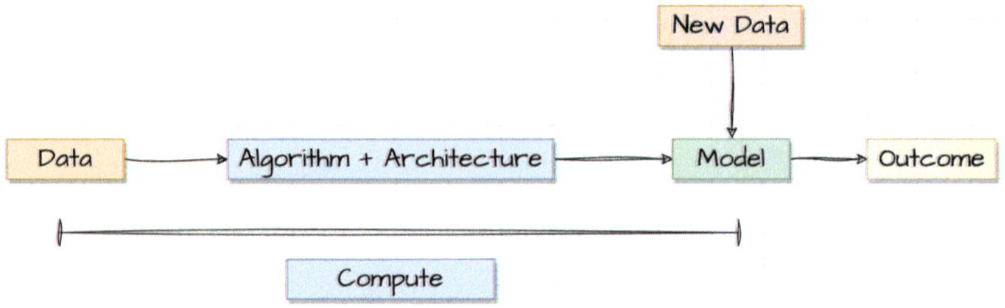

Fig. 4.1 Mental model for artificial intelligence

healthcare challenges through their underlying architecture, purpose, and data requirements (Fig. 4.1).

Components of Artificial Intelligence

Let's start with compute. Compute is analogous to the brain as it is responsible for the processing of the input data [3]. This requires memory to temporarily store the data, and processing power to manipulate the data according to the instructions given to it by the algorithm. It also needs network connectivity to even get the data into the system. All these things make up the compute of AI, and it is the advances in compute that have pushed AI into the spotlight.

However, it is important to emphasize how fundamental processing power is for compute. This is where computer chips enter the picture. Most of us have central processing units, or CPU chips, in our computers which manage all the general instructions required by the operating system and the software that runs on the computer. In AI, there are specialized chips that are especially good at supporting the heavy data processing required which are called graphics processing units, or GPUs [4]. In addition to CPUs and GPUs, companies like Google and Amazon have made even more specialized chips that accommodate specific AI frameworks and specific AI uses that enable the processor to perform faster, and more efficiently [5].

Finally, energy consumption is an important issue for compute. A study by Goldman Sachs, determined that a single query of ChatGPT, which is a special AI example covered in Chap. 5, requires 10 times the electricity than the same query using Google [6]. In fact, they estimate that data center power demands will increase by 160% by 2030 due to the increasing demand for AI, particularly Generative AI. This demand could impact global resources, which is why most cloud service providers have met or are striving to meet the goal of using 100% renewable energies for their data centers. This is also the reason many companies are innovating to make computer chips more energy efficient and less power hungry. It is true that without compute AI would never have happened, but it is equally true that without good, representative data, AI would be limited in its usefulness. Data is the first, and most important, step in the process of building accurate models. Without good data, the model's predictions will be inaccurate.

It is critical to be aware of the standard process that data scientists, and machine learning engineers (henceforth referred to as ML engineers) use to train models. They always start with the data. Data preparation and transformation make up the bulk of their work. ML engineers know that inadequate data quality can undermine their results so they meticulously evaluate each variable to address missing values (imputation), scaling issues which could unfairly weigh one factor over another (normalization & standardization), and sampling methods to ensure there is proper balance of events in the data (class imbalance) [7]. After data prep, they perform feature engineering, which is a term that describes the process of creating new variables from existing ones, or de novo, to enhance performance of the model. An example would be changing a date variable into a day of the week variable. Once they have developed the right algorithm to get the data where they want it, they select their method of implementation (architecture), and then split the data between a training and test samples. They train the model using the training dataset and then test model performance with a new dataset to determine its accuracy. They do this because they want to see how the model will perform with different data, which is also known as generalizability. If a model does not perform well, then it is not generalizable to other data, and as a result is less effective. This is akin to the medical student who memorizes the textbook description of the clinical signs and symptoms of a disease (their mental model of the disease) only to learn the patient they are evaluating hasn't read the book because they have signs and symptoms that don't fit neatly into that mental model. Overreliance on the training data (or the textbook in our analogy) is called 'overfitting' the model in AI parlance, and not having a robust enough model is 'underfitting' [8]. Both will lead to a model that does not provide a good, accurate outcome.

Another important aspect to discuss is the variety of data. We live in a multimodal world where we are inundated with audio, video, and text. Each of these data types require a different algorithm and architectural approach, and different preprocessing methods to prepare the data for analysis. If a problem required unstructured text (such as clinical notes), then there will be a different approach needed to extract that text before the AI system can provide insights. The special area of AI called Natural Language Processing uses AI to do just that—extract data trapped in digital documents so that it can be used by digital systems [9]. Often, the ML engineer will need to use multiple data types to accomplish the goal of a project. Take, as an example, a radiological assessment study that identifies single pulmonary nodules on chest computerized tomography (CT) examinations. The chest CT images would require AI that processes images and identifies patterns in the data, but it will also require text extraction of the radiological report to determine the gold standard result (or outcome label) to determine whether the predictions from the image processing algorithm are correct or not [10]. Without these two different forms of data, the project would require manual labeling of data, which would be more time-consuming.

The potential dangers data can bring to AI models are manifold. One of the biggest concerns with AI is bias. Bias is inherently a data problem because AI algorithms are extremely good at recognizing patterns in the data. If there is a pattern that results from some sort of systematic bias, then the algorithm can make predictions and recommendations that are also biased [11]. Many of the AI platforms and frameworks have developed ways to evaluate for, and mitigate bias, but if the ML engineer is not making bias evaluation a priority it can still become an issue. See Chap. 10 for more about biases in AI applications.

Another challenge, especially for healthcare, is transparency. Many AI systems are considered 'black box' systems, which means it is not easily discernible how the output was derived from the input data, or another way of saying it is that it is not easily explainable [12]. We will dive into this more after we've talked about the different architectures used for deep learning models, and when we wrap up the chapter in the challenges and limitations section.

The next components, algorithms and architectures, have a symbiotic relationship. An algorithm is a set of steps the computer follows to accomplish a desired outcome. This is true of everyday life as well—in the kitchen we call it a recipe, and in medicine we call it a protocol or clinical practice guideline. But algorithms do not operate in isolation; they interact closely with the other components already discussed. For example, an algorithm helps shape the data as previously described, and it interacts with the architecture of the system to optimize how compute is used. Ultimately, all these components work together to create a model. An architecture is a component that serves as a bridge between the compute and algorithm. The architecture often determines how algorithms interact with the compute and can determine how the model learns when processing the data. The interdependence of these components is demonstrated by the fact that the compute you use (CPUs, GPUs, etc.)—can limit what algorithms and architectures can be used, and vice versa [5].

As with data, there are a wide variety of algorithms. Each one suited to solve different problems. So, how do you select the right algorithm? The first critical step is to understand what you are trying to accomplish. Most often, this comes down to what is your outcome variable of interest. Are you analyzing non contrast CT images of the brain to classify the subtypes of intracranial hemorrhage (ICH)? [13] Or, are you using structured clinical trial (cohort) data to forecast a patient's risk of having a cardiovascular event in the next 10 years [14]? The former is a classification outcome, and the latter is a prediction outcome. The next consideration is the type of data you are using (complexity, size, etc.). In the case of the ICH study, they used a large, complex, image repository (one million images from over 25,000 CT scans) which required significant processing power (1 CPU, and 4 GPUs). To handle the grid-based structure of image data, they used an architecture called Convolutional Neural Networks (CNNs). This architecture is particularly well-suited for image classification tasks. CNNs are typically trained using learning algorithms like backpropagation and other adaptive learning optimizers that we'll explore more in the next section [15]. Additionally, they employed another architectural component called Recurrent Neural Networks (RNNs), which are ideal for processing sequential or time-series data [16]. In this study, the RNN architecture helped analyze the series of images in each CT scan. To better understand how these different architectural components work together, we need to dive deeper into the overall architecture of neural networks. (Fig. 4.2).

Inspired by the biological neuron, a neural network (NN) is a computational structure that is composed of interconnected nodes, or neurons, that are organized in parallel layers. These layers are categorized as the input layer, the output layer, and the hidden layers (middle layers). Each connected neuron has a weight which determines its overall importance to the network. The more hidden layers that are present, the 'deeper' the neural network. This distinction will be discussed more when we compare machine learning versus deep learning methods (Fig. 4.3).

The network processes data by passing data from the input layer through the hidden layers to the output layer. At each neuron, the incoming signals are combined, modified by an activation function which converts the inputs into a single output, and then passes it on to the next layer. As the model is trained, the network adjusts its weights to improve its performance on a given task, such as image recognition or language translation. This ability to learn from data and adjust its internal parameters makes neural networks powerful tools, and accounts for the improved performance and accuracy over time with more and more training.

The final point to be made about architecture is that the word *architecture* can also represent the design of an overall AI system rather than just one component. The term that reflects a more complicated design, as found in the Zhang, et al. ICH study, is ensemble methods. Ensemble methods involve using multiple algorithms together to produce the desired results [17]. In the Zhang ICH study, they used a CNN to determine the features of the images that were consistent with an intracranial hemorrhage, which was an important first step, and then fed those results into two RNNs for refinement. This approach was taken to simulate the workflow of a radiologist when they evaluate neuroimaging to determine if a patient has an intracranial hemorrhage. Just as a radiologist might first identify key image features and then consider them in the context of the full scan series, this ensemble architecture

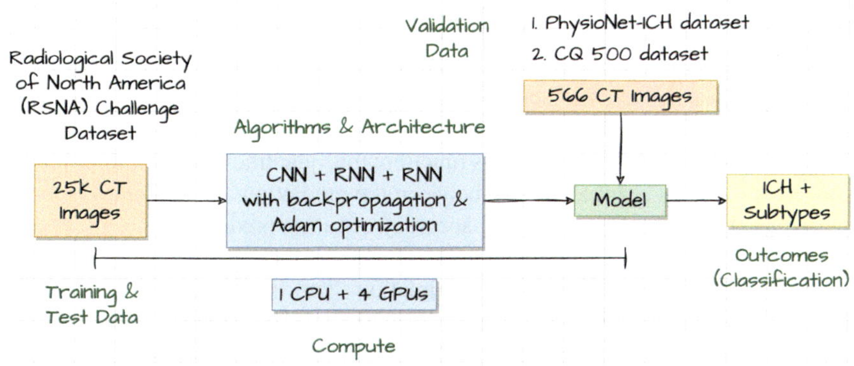

Fig. 4.2 Mental model for Zhang, et al. ICH study

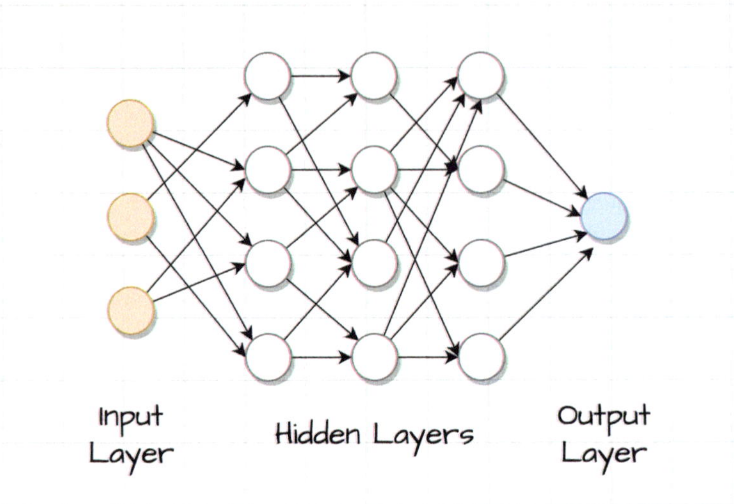

Fig. 4.3 Neural network

processes image features (via CNN) and then analyzes them in sequence (via RNNs). The ultimate goal of artificial intelligence is the creation of a model that makes accurate predictions when analyzing new data. This could be a prediction of what the next word is going to be in a string of text as in the case of Generative AI, or whether the patient sitting in your office is at risk of having a cardiac event in the next 10 years. It's important to recognize that the model is only possible when the architecture and algorithm uses the training data to create the model weights. These model weights are critical to the learning and improvement by the model and require a more in-depth look at the algorithmic learning methods.

While a model is learning, especially one built by neural networks, it's essentially trying to find the best way to make accurate predictions. This is called optimization [18]. It's similar to a cardiac sonographer adjusting the gain on the ultrasound to get the clearest image of the heart during an echocardiogram. These adjustments of the model weights are accomplished with different methods. One method as mentioned in the Zhang ICH study is backpropagation. This is primarily used by neural networks and is a method that adjusts weights by working backwards from the outcome. The computer tracks the gap between the prediction and the actual outcome by something called the loss function; this quantifies the error in its prediction. As it learns, it reduces the gap between the prediction and outcome (reducing the size of the error), it improves the accuracy of future predictions.

Another optimization mentioned in the Zhang, et al's ICH study is Adam, which is shorthand for Adaptive Moment Estimation. The investigators analyzed over 25,000 CT scans for intracranial hemorrhage, the model needed to learn to recognize subtle patterns in the images that indicate bleeding. The Adam optimizer helped this learning process by continuously adjusting the model's internal parameters to improve its ability to detect hemorrhages, while tracking how these adjustments affect the model's accuracy. For instance, Adam might identify that adjustments to the parameters responsible for detecting subtle density changes in brain tissue are consistently improving performance. In response, Adam would allow larger, more confident adjustments in this area. Conversely, if changes to parameters dealing with bone structure recognition aren't helping much, Adam would make smaller, more cautious adjustments there. This adaptive approach helps the model quickly focus on the most relevant image features for hemorrhage detection, potentially leading to faster training and better accuracy in identifying different types of intracranial bleeds, even subtle ones that might be challenging to spot consistently. These are just two of the many techniques AI can use when helping the model improve with data over time.

Other factors influencing model performance include the decisions made regarding the learning process. These choices are called hyperparameters and are usually made during algorithm creation [19]. Examples include how quickly the model should learn (learning rate), how much data it should look at each time it updates its model weights (batch size), and how complex the model structure should be (number of layers in a neural network). Choosing these settings well is crucial for the model to learn effectively and produce reliable results. Often these hyperparameters also need to be adjusted, as with the model weights, to optimize learning. This process is known as hyperparameter tuning and can be done in an automated fashion in some cases. Automated tuning is particularly useful as it can efficiently explore a wide range of combinations, finding optimal settings that might be missed through manual adjustment [19].

Determining if an AI model is ready for real-world use involves several key measurements to evaluate its performance. Machine learning engineers assess how well the model is learning by examining its loss function, which as previously indicated is the discrepancy between the model's predictions and the correct outcomes. For classification tasks, they consider the model's overall accuracy (how often it is correct), precision (the reliability of its positive predictions), and recall (its ability to identify all positive cases). They also use the F1 score, which balances precision and recall. Additionally, the Area Under the Receiver Operating Curve (AUC-ROC) is used to assess how well the model distinguishes between different categories. For regression tasks, measures like the mean absolute error (average size of errors) are utilized. Importantly, the model is tested on both familiar data and new data to ensure it generalizes well. What constitutes "good enough" performance varies depending on the model's intended application, how it compares to existing methods of human performance, and the potential impact of errors in that specific context [20]. Having examined AI's core components, let's now explore how AI systems are classified into distinct but often overlapping categories. As illustrated in Fig. 4.4, these classifications form a hierarchical structure that helps us understand the relationships between different AI capabilities.

AI is the term used for all AI technologies. It is a broad term with no specificity. Machine learning encompasses methods by which the machine learns from the data. Deep learning is a special subset of machine learning and denotes the use of deep neural networks as we discussed briefly in the neural network section of this

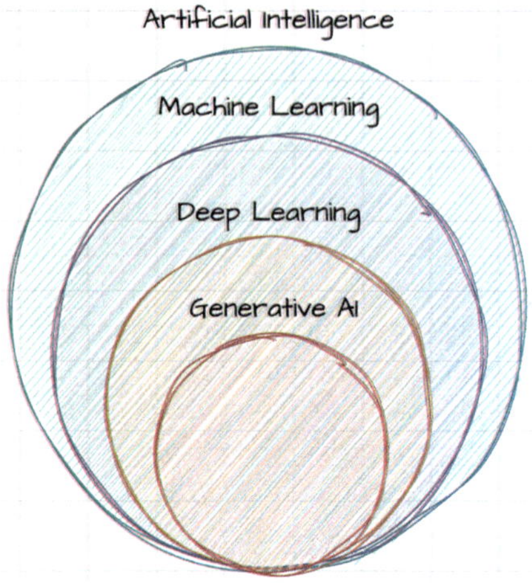

Fig. 4.4 Subtypes of artificial intelligence

chapter. Finally, Generative AI is a special subset of deep learning that will be discussed in more depth in its own dedicated chapter.

Machine Learning

Machine learning has three subtypes: supervised learning, unsupervised learning, and reinforcement learning [21]. The distinctions between these subtypes lie in the way the models are trained, and the ultimate goals of each learning type. With supervised learning, the models are trained on labeled data (also known as the 'ground truth', usually determined by a subject matter expert). The ultimate goal of supervised learning is predicting future outcomes. Unsupervised learning, on the other hand, works with unlabeled data with the aim of uncovering hidden patterns in the data (Fig. 4.5).

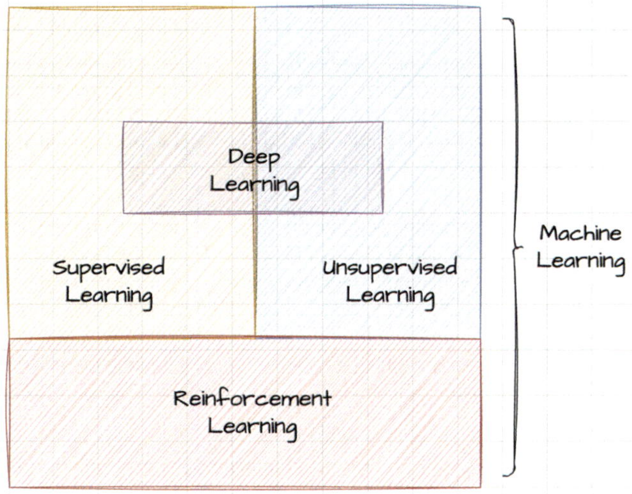

Fig. 4.5 Subtypes of machine learning

Deep Learning

Deep learning refers to machine learning that uses neural networks that have many (>3) hidden layers. But as is implied in the definition, neural networks that have less than 3 layers are considered shallow networks and would not meet the criteria for deep learning [22].

Another key distinction between traditional machine learning and deep learning is their approach to feature extraction and model complexity. In ML, features often need to be manually engineered or selected by domain experts, requiring significant human input to determine which aspects of the data are most relevant for the task at hand. This process relies heavily on expertise and intuition. ML models, such as decision trees, support vector machines, or shallow neural networks, then use these pre-defined features to make predictions or classifications. In contrast, DL models are capable of automatically learning relevant features from raw data through their multiple layers of processing. This automatic feature extraction is one of the key strengths of DL, allowing it to discover complex patterns that might not be apparent to human experts, especially in high-dimensional data like images or speech.

Deep learning techniques are used in supervised learning as well as unsupervised learning. A prominent example of deep learning used in supervised learning is Convolutional Neural Networks. CNNs, as discussed earlier in the Zhang, et al. ICH study, are particularly effective for image classification tasks.

Other examples where CNNs have been used in healthcare are: diagnosing diabetic retinopathy from retinal images, detecting lung nodules in chest X-rays, classifying skin lesions as benign or malignant from dermatological images, and identifying brain tumors on MRI scans.

Table 4.1 Machine learning outcomes & methods

ML Types	Outcomes	Methods (Limited List)
Supervised	Predicting Continuous Values (like Percent, or Cost) Classifying into Categories (like High Risk of Stroke, Intermediate Risk of Stroke, and Low Risk of Stroke, or like blood types: A, B, AB, and O)	Regression Models Tree Based Models Support Vector Machines (SVM) Neural Networks Bayesian Methods Ensemble Methods Boosting Methods
Unsupervised	Grouping Similar Items Reducing Data Complexity Detecting Unusual Items Finding hidden patterns Generating new data	K-means Clustering Hierarchical Clustering Principal Component Analysis One Class SVM Variational Autoendcoders Generative Adversarial Neural Networks (GANs)
Reinforcement	Improved Decision-Making Efficient Strategies Learned Behaviors	Q-Learning Deep Q-Networks (DQN) Policy Gradient Methods

In these examples, the CNN is trained on a large dataset of labeled images (supervision). The network learns to recognize relevant features, such as edges, textures, and more complex patterns, in the images and associates them with the correct labels. Once trained, it can classify new, unlabeled images. Finally, the third subtype of machine learning is Reinforcement Learning. With Reinforcement Learning, the goal is to train an agent (a car, toy, robot, trading bot, or gaming character to name a few) that gets rewarded or penalized with each decision to maximize reward accumulation [23]. In other words, it is not trained by labeled data or to look for patterns, but instead to make good decisions. The agent is given a set of rules for rewards and penalties with the objective for the agent to score the highest points possible. Reinforcement Learning is about learning optimal strategies through trial and error (Table 4.1).

Applications of AI in Healthcare

The following are practical examples of supervised learning, unsupervised learning, deep learning and reinforcement learning from the medical literature.

Supervised Learning The Framingham Heart Study began in 1948 after Harry Truman signed the National Heart Act into law. This act was part of a broader effort to address the high rates of cardiovascular disease in the United States, an issue highlighted by the death of Franklin Delano Roosevelt from hypertensive stroke. This landmark cohort study helped establish the risk factors now known to be responsible for cardiovascular deaths [24].

Let's imagine the original dataset looked something like the table below. Each variable would have a value per participant in the study, and when you look at the algorithm used (regression model) to analyze all the variables, you would be able to determine each factor's impact (weight) on the model. These weights are known as

Table 4.2 Example dataset from Framingham Heart Study

Patient	CVD outcome	Blood pressure	Smoker	Total cholesterol
1	Yes	140/89	Yes	220
2	No	120/70	No	160
3	No	100/75	No	140
4	Yes	168/100	Yes	195
5	Yes	145/99	No	175

regression coefficients. The labeled data point is the cardiovascular disease (CVD) outcome, which is used to determine the accuracy of all future predictions based on the other data points in the dataset (Table 4.2).

The Framingham Risk Score uses these regression coefficients to calculate (or predict) future cardiovascular risk over the next decade. This is a simple model, but it is a great example of how supervised learning, which has been traditionally used most in clinical trials, contributes to the everyday practice of medicine. The additional benefit of using this simple model is the explainability of the model.

Unsupervised Learning

The Swedish ANDIS (All New Diabetics in Scania) study was a large scale, cohort study that began in 2008 where over 20,000 new diabetics were followed over a decade for the purpose of studying diabetes heterogeneity [25]. Using easily available clinical data such as A1C, Body Mass Index, Date of diabetes onset, Glutamate Decarboxylase Autoantibodies (GADA), C-peptide, and several other factors, a cluster analysis was performed that identified 5 subtypes in the cohort: Insulin Deficient, Insulin Resistance, Obesity Related, Later Age Onset, and Severe Autoimmune Diabetes (SAID). This study highlights how using unsupervised learning, k-means & hierarchical cluster analysis, can identify patterns in the data as was found with these 5 distinct subtypes. This study suggested the potential to personalize treatment for each subtype and challenged the notion of defining a disease with a single metabolite such as glucose.

Deep Learning

To demonstrate a powerful example of a deep learning study, we return to the Intracranial Hemorrhage study [13]. The study was performed in 2021 with the purpose of evaluating a deep learning algorithm's ability to detect and classify acute intracranial hemorrhage (ICH) on head CT scans. The researchers employed a multi-stage approach combining a 2D convolutional neural network and two recurrent neural networks. The model was trained using over 25,000 CT scans from the 2019 RSNA

Brain CT Hemorrhage Challenge dataset, with further validation on two independent external datasets: PhysioNet-ICH (75 scans) and CQ500 (491 scans). On the RSNA test set, the algorithm achieved an impressive AUC of 0.988 for overall ICH detection, with AUCs for ICH subtypes ranging from 0.983 to 0.996. Performance remained high on the external datasets, with AUCs of 0.964 and 0.949 for overall ICH detection. The algorithm outperformed previous methods in the literature and matched expert radiologist performance. Key lessons from the study include the benefits of incorporating 3D context information (the RNNs), the algorithm's ability to generalize well across different imaging protocols and patient populations, and the use of saliency maps to enhance interpretability. The researchers concluded that their method could potentially serve as a valuable second-read or triage tool in clinical practice, though they emphasized the need for further validation before deployment.

Reinforcement Learning

There have been many retrospective observational studies using reinforcement learning for protocol adherence with simulated outcomes [26]. Many of these were studied in ICU settings where researchers evaluated sepsis treatment policies, mechanical ventilation management, and even HIV treatment using CD4+ T-cell counts to adjust treatment regimens [27, 28]. The studies generally show promise with better outcomes and improved protocol adherence with RL but given the nature of the real time data and adjustment requirements, and the high-risk nature of these subject areas, it is highly likely this area of research will progress slowly, and with great caution as it should. This naturally transitions to our final section where we discuss limitations and challenges.

Conclusion

AI can produce powerful tools to support clinicians when caring for patients. However, the clinician must understand the basics of AI, as well as its limitations and benefits, in order to champion its appropriate use for future patient care.

Limitations and Challenges of AI

In the daily practice of medicine, risk and benefits are evaluated, or should be, with each intervention decision made. I would posit AI should be no different. However, this will take intentionality by clinicians and by regulatory agencies as many times AI can be embedded into systems that abstract away its reliance from the clinician.

So what are the risks of using AI? Here we'll share a list of considerations but it should not be considered all encompassing because it is certainly possible new ones will arise in the future.

One of the biggest risks in healthcare has always been data security and privacy as acknowledged by the enactment of the Health Insurance Portability and Accountability Act in 1996. Back then, it was all about managing paper records, but today it is an even bigger challenge with the ease of portability of electronic records. The risk is compounded by the use of the patient's records to train models if the models are not sufficiently secured. There have been numerous instances where bad actors have stolen records from healthcare systems, and this will be a challenge with future AI models, especially language models, if not addressed.

Another challenge with AI was uncovered in 1997 when Cooper et al. performed a study using machine learning to predict mortality in patients with pneumonia [29]. The goal was to provide a model that could predict the patients who had a high probability of death. This could help ambulatory clinicians admit the high risk patients to reduce mortality from pneumonia. They used a neural net to evaluate the data and found that the neural net outperformed the logistic regression model by a large margin (AUC 0.86 versus 0.77). The only problem was that when they looked at the data and the rules the neural net created from the data—they noted that the neural net predicted patients with asthma had a lower risk of mortality. As they dug into the data used by the neural net for training, they realized that the patients with asthma were actually hospitalized more often than non asthmatics in favor of aggressive treatment, and as a result had a lower mortality than the non asthmatic group. This highlighted the need to explainability of the results when using AI, which led to them championing the concept of intelligible machine learning models.

Unfortunately, mistakes, and bad outcomes, are part of medicine. And though no one ever wants harm to come to a patient, it still happens. The question is rarely who is responsible. That question is usually very clear from the medical record of who provided the care for the patient. However, what if the mistake occurred as a result of what an AI model recommended? What if the clinician dutifully executed the recommendation made by the system and that recommendation was flawed? Who is responsible? The clinician or the system that led the clinician astray? These are the future issues healthcare will need to address before there is wide implementation of AI systems.

Finally, we could talk about the ethics of using AI that has not been proven (in other words experimental), the lack of consent to use patient data for training AI models, the risk of disparities in care based on biased training data used by AI systems, and much, much more. The important thread that weaves through all these issues that the healthcare community needs to be involved and engaged to ensure we champion the use of AI that is responsible, ethical, and humane. We need to be the bridge between the technical advancements and the implementation in our practices.

References

1. RBC Capital Markets. Navigating the changing face of healthcare. Available at: https://www.rbccm.com/en/gib/healthcare/episode/the_healthcare_data_explosion. Accessed 5 Oct 2024.
2. HealthTech. Structured vs. unstructured data in healthcare. Available at: https://healthtechmagazine.net/article/2020/07/structured-vs-unstructured-data-healthcare. Accessed 5 Oct 2024.
3. Rajkumar. Central Processing Unit (CPU): The brain of the computer. Software testing material. Published August 11, 2024. Available at: https://www.softwaretestingmaterial.com/cpu-brain-of-the-computer. Accessed 5 Oct 2024.
4. Reznik A, Nelson T, Abdo K, Xu C. Why GPUs are essential for AI and high-performance computing. Red Hat Developer. Published November 21, 2022. Available at: https://developers.redhat.com/articles/why-gpus-are-essential-ai-and-high-performance-computing. Accessed 5 Oct 2024.
5. Pynomial. AI Chips Overview: TPU, NPU, GPU, and FPGA. Published 2023. Available at: https://pynomial.com/ai-chips-overview. Accessed 5 Oct 2024.
6. Goldman Sachs Research. AI's impact on power consumption: ChatGPT vs. Google Search. USGI. Published June 3, 2024. Available at: https://www.usfunds.com. Accessed 5 Oct 2024.
7. Intelliarts. Data preparation in machine learning: 6 steps guide. Available at: https://intelliarts.com. Accessed 5 Oct 2024.
8. Artificial Intelligence School. A guide to overfitting and underfitting in machine learning. Available at: https://artificialintelligenceschool.com. Accessed 5 Oct 2024.
9. ibml. Role of artificial intelligence in document digitization. Available at: https://www.ibml.com. Accessed 5 Oct 2024.
10. Caruana R, Koch P, Lou Y, et al. Intelligible models for healthcare: predicting pneumonia risk and hospital 30-day readmission. In: Proceedings of the 21st ACM SIGKDD international conference on knowledge discovery and data mining. ACM; 2015. p. 1721–30.
11. World Economic Forum. Research shows AI is often biased. Here's how to make algorithms work for all of us. Available at: https://www.weforum.org. Accessed 5 Oct 2024.
12. University of Michigan-Dearborn. AI's mysterious 'black box' problem, explained. Available at: https://umdearborn.edu. Accessed 5 Oct 2024.
13. Zhang J, Han X, Wang X, et al. A deep learning algorithm for automatic detection and classification of acute intracranial hemorrhages in head CT scans. NeuroImage Clin. 2021;31:102785.
14. Goff DC Jr, Lloyd-Jones DM, Bennett G, Coady S, D'Agostino RB, Gibbons R, et al. 2013 ACC/AHA guideline on the assessment of cardiovascular risk: a report of the American College of Cardiology/American Heart Association Task Force on Practice Guidelines. Circulation. 2014;129(25 Suppl 2):S49–73.
15. Aytaç UC, Güneş A, Ajlouni N. A novel adaptive momentum method for medical image classification using convolutional neural network. BMC Med Imaging. 2022;22(1):34.
16. Amazon Web Services. What is a recurrent neural network? Available at: https://aws.amazon.com/what-is/recurrent-neural-network/. Accessed 5 Oct 2024.
17. IBM. Ensemble learning: what is ensemble learning? Available at: https://www.ibm.com/topics/ensemble-learning. Accessed 5 Oct 2024.
18. Chen J, Liu Y. Neural optimization machine: a neural network approach for optimization. Arxiv.org/2208.03897v1.
19. Amazon Web Services. What is hyperparameter tuning? Available at: https://aws.amazon.com/what-is/hyperparameter-tuning/. Accessed 5 Oct 2024.
20. Fiddler AI. Which is more important: model performance or model accuracy? Available at: https://www.fiddler.ai/model-accuracy-vs-model-performance/which-is-more-important-model-performance-or-model-accuracy. Accessed 5 Oct 2024.
21. IBM. Types of machine learning. Available at: https://www.ibm.com/think/topics/machine-learning-types. Accessed 5 Oct 2024.

22. McKinsey & Company. What is deep learning? Available at: https://www.mckinsey.com/what-is-deep-learning. Accessed 5 Oct 2024.
23. MarkTechPost. Reinforcement learning: training AI agents through rewards and penalties. Available at: https://www.marktechpost.com. Accessed 5 Oct 2024.
24. Abohelwa M, Kopel J, Shurmur S, Ansari MM, Awasthi Y, Awasthi S. The Framingham study on cardiovascular disease risk and stress-defenses: a historical review. J Vasc Dis. 2023;2(1):122–64. Available at: https://www.mdpi.com. Accessed 5 Oct 2024.
25. Groop L. All New Diabetics in Scania (ANDIS). Swedish National Data Service. Published 2008. Available at: https://snd.se. Accessed 5 Oct 2024.
26. Lauffenburger JC, Yom-Tov E, Keller PA, et al. REinforcement learning to improve non-adherence for diabetes treatments by Optimising Response and Customising Engagement (REINFORCE): study protocol of a pragmatic randomised trial. Trials. 2023; Available at: https://bmjopen.bmj.com. Accessed 5 Oct 2024.
27. Saria S. Individualized sepsis treatment using reinforcement learning. Nat Med. 2018;24(11):1641–2.
28. Raghu A, Komorowski M, Celi LA, Szolovits P, Ghassemi M. Continuous state-space models for optimal sepsis treatment: a deep reinforcement learning approach. Mach Learn Healthc Conf Proc. 2017;68:147–63.
29. Cooper GF, Aliferis CF, Ambrosino R, et al. An evaluation of machine-learning methods for predicting pneumonia mortality. Artif Intell Med. 1997;9(2):107–38.

Chapter 5
Generative Artificial Intelligence

David Carnahan

Introduction

In the fall of 2022, OpenAI released a generative spark that set the world ablaze with a simple chatbot called ChatGPT. Within 5 days, there were one million users, and within 2 months, there were over 100 million [1]. It was the fastest adoption of a new technology of its kind. What has followed has been nothing short of remarkable. Large Tech companies, Meta, Amazon, Microsoft, Google, and many others, have invested heavily in generative AI because of its future potential to improve customers daily lives.

As mentioned in Chap. 4, Generative Artificial Intelligence (Gen AI) is a subset of Deep Learning. It is a special brand of AI that generates new output based on instructions, data, and algorithms. The input can be text, images, or both, and can produce anything from text, to images, to voice, and even video. The variety of output has captured the imaginations of industries from healthcare, education, computer science, business, and arts and entertainment.

This chapter covers the components of Gen AI, the process it uses to generate new content, the different ways application developers try to harness it while eliminating hallucinations and inaccurate results, and how it can help healthcare. Finally, this chapter will cover, as before, the challenges and limitations to consider when using Gen AI. To reduce the complexity of the discussion, this chapter will focus solely on text based Generative AI.

This chapter does not represent the views of AWS.

D. Carnahan (✉)
Amazon Web Services, Worldwide Public Sector, San Antonio, TX, USA

T. Adirim (ed.), *Digital Health, AI and Generative AI in Healthcare*,
https://doi.org/10.1007/978-3-031-83526-1_5

Components of Generative AI

The components for Generative AI are similar to those discussed in Chap. 4 on AI fundamentals with the exception that there are notable differences in the algorithms and architecture. To recap, all AI needs compute, data, algorithms, architectures, and models. Machine Learning experts use compute to process data, which generally uses data specific architectures and algorithms to build a model. This model then predicts the outcomes of interest when fed new data based on what it has learned from the training data.

Compute

Generative AI requires a lot of processing, almost exclusively from graphic processing units (GPU). This is due to the amount of data needed to train Large Language Models (LLMs). These models engage in complicated calculations to generate new content. For these reasons LLMs require clusters of GPUs, which means GPUs are connected so that they can operate as a unified system [2]. In fact, in March of 2023, a research firm, TrendForce, estimated ChatGPT would need up to 30,000 GPUs to power its LLM [3]. This would be equivalent to connecting 40,000 to 50,000 laptop computers together so you can use the combined compute power as if it were one supercomputer. Earlier in 2024, Meta announced plans to invest in 350,000 Nvidia GPUs for its work to create human-like intelligence, also known as Artificial General Intelligence (AGI) [4]. So, the biggest difference between the compute needed for general AI and Generative is the scale required.

Data

Without data, there is no model. But what kind of data is needed for LLMs, and how much? Most LLM developers train their model on all the data they can get their hands on. In fact, Google famously agreed to pay $60 million dollars a year for Reddit data to train its models [5]. Another example of the magnitude of data used to train LLMs is found with the models Meta released. In their first version of Llama, they reportedly used 1.4 trillion tokens to train the model. The second release used two trillion tokens, and the most recent, Llama 3, used 15 trillion tokens to train the model [6].

The data used to train LLMs includes a large body of text (also called corpus) obtained from all the websites on the internet known as the Common Crawler [7]. This repository of data is freely available to everyone. The organization managing the repository has been crawling the internet since 2007, and the repository is reported to contain over 250 billion websites with 3–5 billion new websites added each month. Each monthly crawl contains petabytes of data. And there are variants of this data—Google, for one example, manages a cleaned version of the Common Crawl that they call the 'Colossal Clean Crawled Corpus' (C4). Another large repository of data is known as The Pile [8]. This data source is a large, diverse, open-source language modeling dataset created by EleutherAI. In total, it contains twenty-two smaller, high-quality datasets such as scientific papers (medical, math, physics, computer science), GitHub repositories, books, webpages, chat logs, and philosophy papers. This data repository is attractive to model builders because it provides reasoning processes in the publications. This theoretically provides the LLMs with the ability to learn reasoning skills from the training data.

However, it is important to understand that many of the corporations who are training LLMs have access to data that the public will never have access to. In fact, this issue of how these corporations may be training their models with this data has provoked many to question the use of private data without consent from the creators of that data. This issue will continue to be one discussed for a long time as creators litigate against perceived improper use of their data. This will be a hard line to reestablish once the model has been already trained on data, but it is one that is important for regulators to detangle in the interest of protecting the intellectual property (art, novels, blogs, etc.) of creators.

Algorithms & Architecture

The Process

Let us dive into the process that Gen AI follows when taking information in the form of a question or command, also known as a prompt, to generate new content. We will focus on the text based generative AI examples rather than image based or multimodal. There will be differences in the process used by all three types of Gen AI output.

The first thing that happens is the generative AI system breaks the prompt down into smaller pieces known as tokens. These tokens could be words, or even parts of words. Then, each token is converted to a vector (or string) of numbers. This numerical representation of the tokens is also known as an embedding [9]. As a side note, this conversion to numbers allows the compute to more easily perform all the processing tasks that will be required of it. The compute then takes the embeddings and determines the context of each token within the prompt and modifies its embedding to provide the context of the prompt. This context will improve the language model ability to return an appropriate response. After this processing, the model predicts the next token to add based on the contextualized prompt. It does this one token at a time until the LLM stops the process. Finally, the compute then provides the response, which it has converted from tokens back to text, to the user as its output [10].

Remarkably, this happens within a fraction of a second. For better understanding, consider the following example:

User Input

"Define stroke."

Tokenization

The input text is broken down into smaller units called tokens.

Tokens: ['Define', 'stroke', '.']

Encoding

Tokens are converted into numerical representations (embeddings) that the model can process.

Contextualization

The model processes these embeddings through multiple layers, understanding relationships and meanings based on prior training. We will discuss this in more detail when we discuss self-attention in the next section.

Encodings: [2184, 9087, 1012]

Contextual Embeddings: [0.8, -1.5, 0.3]

Prediction

The model generates a response by predicting the next token based on the contextualized prompt. The predicted embedding is then converted to a token. This process happens iteratively, one token at a time, until the model comes to the end of the response.

Predicted Embeddings: [0.9, -1.0, 1.2, ...]

Predicted Tokens: ['A', 'stroke', 'is', 'a', 'medical', 'condition', 'that', 'occurs', 'when', 'the', 'blood', 'supply', 'to', 'part', 'of', 'the', 'brain', 'is', 'interrupted', 'or', 'reduced', ',', 'preventing', 'brain', 'tissue', 'from', 'getting', 'oxygen', 'and', 'nutrients', '.']

Decoding

The numerical representations (predicted embeddings) are converted back into tokens, and then readable text.

Decoded Text: "A stroke is a medical condition that occurs when the blood supply to part of the brain is interrupted or reduced, preventing brain tissue from getting oxygen and nutrients."

Output

The final text is provided as the response to the user's input.

Model Output: "A stroke is a medical condition that occurs when the blood supply to part of the brain is interrupted or reduced, preventing brain tissue from getting oxygen and nutrients."

Transformers & Self-Attention

In this section, we will dive deeper into the process above to provide the proper context for the prompt. To do this, we need to discuss transformers. In 2017, Google Engineers released an open scientific paper titled "Attention is All You Need" [11]. In the paper, they addressed one of the biggest challenges for Gen AI up to that point—context. This paper proposed using a new architecture, the transformer, and a self-attention algorithm which provided the innovative spark needed to push the field of Gen AI forward.

What is a transformer? Technically speaking, a transformer is a neural network architecture that uses its layers to map an input sequence (prompt) to an output sequence. It does this by leveraging the self-attention algorithm to capture relationships between tokens. The process we reviewed earlier is the way transformers accomplish the mapping.

Self-attention enables the model to focus on all the different tokens of the input at the same time. It does this by computing the relevance of each token to every other input token, which captures the complex relationships within the input sequence. The mechanism works in parallel across tokens using the transformer's attention layers (hidden neural network layers), which provides significant efficiency.

Once the relationships of the tokens to each other are established, the self-attention mechanism incorporates these relationships into the embeddings for each token. It does this by modifying the embedding, mathematically, for each token to include the context of how it is used in the prompt. This context-aware representation is crucial for generating contextually appropriate outputs.

Predictions

The whole point of the mathematical gymnastics that transformers use is to get a good prediction of what the next token should be. As the transformer processes the input sequence through its layers, it refines, transforms, and processes the data to determine a collection of the most likely next words, which are then provided as output [10].

This contextualization allows for greater understanding of what is being asked of the model, and as the output is generated, each new token is added to the input sequence to update the context. This improves the accuracy of the selection/ of the next token. It does this until the model terminates the sequence.

Encoder-Decoder

The encoder-decoder architecture, described in our example, functions as a two-part machine for processing language. The encoder takes in a sentence and analyzes it thoroughly. It creates a deep understanding of its meaning and context. The decoder takes this understanding and uses it to generate a new sentence, one word at a time. Importantly, while the decoder is creating its new sentence, it checks back with the encoder's understanding to make sure it is staying on track.

This back-and-forth between understanding (encoding) and generating (decoding) allows the system to perform complex tasks all while maintaining the original meaning and context of the prompt.

Models

What is a Large Language Model? The answer is in the name—a LLM is a model built with large datasets that learns to understand and interpret human language. These models are commonly used for summarization, language translation, text generation, and question answering [12].

Parameters

If you have been following the releases of the different LLMs (ChatGPT, Claude, Llama, etc.), you probably noticed there has been a flurry of activity ever since the first release of ChatGPT. But what is most interesting is that with each new release comes a significant increase in the number of parameters of the model [13] (Table 5.1).

There is clearly a pattern of increasing complexity of the model as defined by number of parameters. At least it sounds complex when you say a model has billions or even trillions of parameters. But what does that mean? And what exactly are these parameters of the model?

To answer these questions, let us return to the neuron. For simplicity's sake, we will consider a smaller neuron to illustrate what a parameter is. Technically, parameters are nothing more than the weights and biases of the model (Fig. 5.1).

A bias is a learned parameter at the neuron level. It is one of the factors that allow the neuron to fine-tune its response to the data it is being trained on to improve the accuracy of the output of the model. The other significant factor is the weight of the neuron connections. A weight defines the strength of the connection between two neurons. It is by these weights that the neural network learns what is most important and what is less important in the data. Over time, like biases, these weights are refined as the model is trained on a large volume of data [14].

So, how many parameters does our simple neural network have? This turns out to be simple math. The first layer of neurons, the input layer, have no biases. They are the intake layer for the data, which then shares the data with the other layers. The connections between the input and hidden layer have (3 neurons × 4 neurons) 12 connections, which means it has 12 weights. The hidden layer has 4 neurons; all of which will have a bias, and there are (4 × 2) 8 connections. So, there are 8 weights for the hidden layer. Finally, there are two neurons in the output layer, which equates to 2 biases (Table 5.2).

Table 5.1 Estimated number of parameters for select LLMs by release version

Model	Version 1	Version 2	Version 3	Version 4
ChatGPT	117 million	1.5 billion	175 billion	1.76 trillion
Claude	60 billion	176 billion	~500 billion	
Llama	13 billion	70 billion	70 billion	

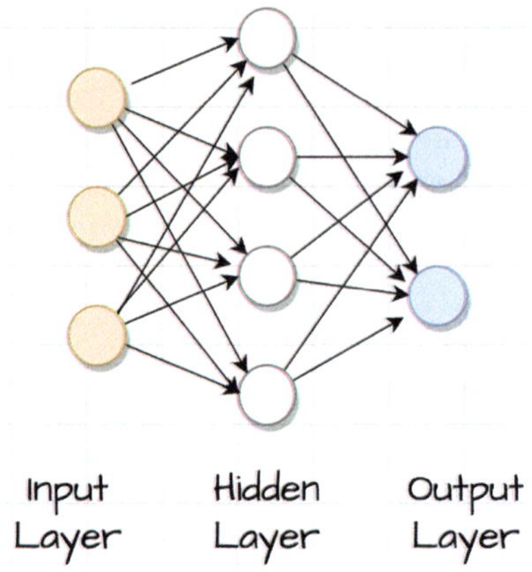

Fig. 5.1 Simple neural network

Table 5.2 Parameter calculations for simple neural network

Layer connection	Bias count	Weight count	Total parameters
Input layer to hidden layer	0	12	12
Hidden layer to output layer	4	8	12
Output layer	2	0	2
Total			26

In sum, you have 26 parameters for this simple neural network. Given this information, you likely deduced that the parameters of the models with billions and trillions of parameters have a LOT of hidden layers in their neural network. You would be right. As a reminder from Chap. 4 on AI fundamentals, the determination of the number of layers along with other settings (learning rate, sample size of data, number of epochs, etc.) used to train LLMs are determined by the hyperparameters of the system.

Model Performance

There are many benchmarks used to evaluate LLM performance. Since LLMs are more complex than routine models used in AI, the metrics of LLM performance are equally more complex. The table below demonstrates the kind of performance metrics LLM developers report when they release a new version of their LLM, which focuses on general knowledge capabilities including graduate level knowledge, math & problem-solving, multilingual problems, computer coding, among other measure domains [15] (Fig. 5.2).

There are many different types of models. The general knowledge LLMs like ChatGPT, Claude, and Llama are often referred to as Foundation Models. As this

	Claude 3.5 Sonnet	Claude 3 Opus	GPT-4o	Gemini 1.5 Pro	Llama-400b (early snapshot)
Graduate level reasoning *GPQA, Diamond*	**59.4%*** 0-shot CoT	**50.4%** 0-shot CoT	**53.6%** 0-shot CoT	---	---
Undergraduate level knowledge *MMLU*	**88.7%**** 5-shot **88.3%** 0-shot CoT	**86.8%** 5-shot **85.7%** 0-shot CoT	--- **88.7%** 0-shot CoT	**85.9%** 5-shot ---	**86.1%** 5-shot ---
Code *HumanEval*	**92.0%** 0-shot	**84.9%** 0-shot	**90.2%** 0-shot	**84.1%** 0-shot	**84.1%** 0-shot
Multilingual math *MGSM*	**91.6%** 0-shot CoT	**90.7%** 0-shot CoT	**90.5%** 0-shot CoT	**87.5%** 8-shot	---
Reasoning over text *DROP, F1score*	**87.1** 3-shot	**83.1** 3-shot	**83.4** 3-shot	**74.9** Variable shots	**83.5** 3-shot Pre-trained model
Mixed evaluations *BIG-Bench-Hard*	**93.1%** 3-shot CoT	**86.8%** 3-shot CoT	---	**89.2%** 3-shot CoT	**85.3%** 3-shot CoT Pre-trained model
Math problem-solving *MATH*	**71.1%** 0-shot CoT	**60.1%** 0-shot CoT	**76.6%** 0-shot CoT	**67.7%** 4-shot	**57.8%** 4-shot CoT
Grade school math *GSM8K*	**96.4%** 0-shot CoT	**95.0%** 0-shot CoT	---	**90.8%** 11-shot	**94.1%** 8-shot CoT

*Claude 3.5 Sonnet scores 67.2% on 5-shot CoT GPQA with maj@32
**Claude 3.5 Sonnet scores 90.4% on MMLU with 5-shot CoT prompting

Fig. 5.2 Example comparison of benchmark performance with Claude 3.5 Sonnet release [16]. *Claude 3.5 Sonnet scores 67.2% on 5-shot CoT GPQA with maj@32. **Claude 3.5 Sonnet scores 90.4% on MMLU with 5-shot CoT prompting

name implies, they can be tailored to specific uses by using external techniques which will be the remaining focus of this chapter. However, it is important to know that not all LLMs are general. Some have been tailored for specific industries by training their models on industry specific data, which means, theoretically, the model will perform much better on tasks, or assignments of that specific field.

In healthcare, we have a unique vocabulary that falls outside the normal vocabulary of general language. So, it makes sense that training an LLM for biomedical and clinical use on medical specific data would improve performance when the LLM is asked to do biomedical and clinical tasks. Listed below are several examples of LLMs that have been specifically trained on the medical domain [17–20] (Table 5.3).

What about the performance of these models for medical expertise? A study conducted in October of 2023 by Abbas et al. found that ChatGPT 4 performed better than the other models of that time when answering multiple choice questions of the Clinical Subject Exam of the National Board of Medical Examiners (NBME) test. This exam covers medicine, pediatrics, family medicine, and ambulatory care domains, and is generally taken by medical students as they transition from classroom learning into clinical rotations in their third and fourth years [21] (Table 5.4).

Table 5.3 Medical LLMs

LLM	Base LLM	Purpose	Training Data	Developer
ClinicalBERT	BERT	Clinical language understanding and tasks	Clinical notes, medical records	MIT & Researchers
PubMedBERT	BERT	Biomedical NLP tasks	PubMed abstracts and full text	Microsoft & Researchers
BEHRT	BERT	EHR analysis, predicting future diagnoses	Electronic Health Records	King's College London
BioGPT	GPT	Biomedical text generation and understanding	Biomedical literature	Microsoft
Med-PaLM2	PaLM	Medical Q&A, clinical decision support	Medical literature, clinical data	Google
Galactica	Custom	Scientific knowledge tasks, including biomedical	Scientific papers, reference material	Meta
BioMegatron	Megatron	Biomedical NLP tasks	Biomedical literature	Nvidia

Table 5.4 Performance of LLMs on NBME clinical subject exam

Model	Performance	Developer
GPT 4	100% (163/163)	OpenAI
Claude	84.7% (138/163)	Anthropic
GPT 3.5	82.2% (134/163)	OpenAI
BARD	75.5% (123/163)	Google

In another study by Singhal et al., researchers evaluated LLMs (PaLM and Flan-PaLM) on medical knowledge [22]. They created a new benchmark, the MultiMedQA, which combined existing medical datasets and a consumer health question dataset. The models achieved state-of-the-art performance on multiple-choice medical exams. However, human evaluation revealed gaps in Flan-PaLM's answers to consumer health questions (Table 5.5).

The limitations of these studies are inherent in the fact that the advancements in the field of Generative AI are outstripping the ability to study the new models and their performance. In fact, a follow-up study by Singhal et al., showed MedPaLM 2 outperformed physicians in their long form answers in 8 of 9 domains evaluated [23]. This study was performed a mere 3–4 months after the original.

Table 5.5 Evaluation (percent) agreement with blinded clinicians & lay participants

Evaluation topic	Clinician (%)	PaLM (%)	Flan-PaLM (%)
Scientific consensus	92.9	92.6	61.9
Inappropriate or incorrect content	1.4	18.7	16.1
Missing content	11.1	15.3	47.6
Extent of possible harm	5.7	5.9	29.7
Likelihood of possible harm	1.3	2.3	19.4
Possibility of bias	1.4	0.8	7.9
Address intent of question[a]	95.9	94.4	90.8
Helpfulness of answer[a]	91.1	80.3	60.6

[a]Analyzed by lay participants

Prompts & Prompt Engineering

Up to this point, we have been focused on the internal process of developing the LLMs, but now we turn outward—to look at the way external processes are used to influence the safety, reliability, and accuracy of LLMs. However, it must be acknowledged that anything that can be used for good can also be used for maleficence. And now, we turn to prompts and prompt engineering.

Prompts are the instructions the user provides to the LLM to perform a task. These prompts have a spectrum of complexity, ranging from a simple question to complicated scripts that advise the LLM on how to process the request. We will get into these scripts a bit more when we discuss Agents later in the chapter.

Most prompts entered by non-technical users for a chatbot ask a simple question or ask the LLM to do a simple task. But, as mentioned before, there is an art and science to prompts, and you can do a lot with prompting to optimize the response you get from the LLM.

The following list is not an all-inclusive list of prompting techniques, but it is a good start. There is a whole specialty field emerging in this work called prompt engineering, which generally involves complex architectures of system-based prompts, guardrails and other methods to constrain and optimize LLMs [24].

Zero-shot prompting is using a prompt that provides no examples for the LLM to follow.

An example:

Input: Classify the following sentence as either positive or negative sentiment. The concert exceeded all my expectations, it was an unforgettable experience.

Few-shot prompting provides a few examples for the LLM to follow. Think of this as limited training for your specific request.

An example:

Input: Classify the following sentence as either positive or negative sentiment.

Example 1:
Sentence: The movie was fantastic. I loved it!
Classification: Positive
Example 2:
Sentence: The service at this restaurant was terrible.
Classification: Negative
Example 3:
Sentence: I am neutral about the new policy changes.
Classification: Neutral
Now classify this:
Sentence: The concert exceeded my expectations. It was an incredible experience.
Classification:

Chain-of-thought prompting is when a prompt is used for complex reasoning capabilities by utilizing intermediate steps that explain the reasoning process.

An example:

Input: The odd numbers in this group add up to an even number: 4, 8, 9, 15, 12, 2, 1.
A: Adding all the odd numbers (9, 15, 1) gives 25. The answer is False.
Input: The odd numbers in this group add up to an even number: 15, 32, 5, 13, 82, 7, 1.
A:

The example of above could also be called **Few-shot Chain-of-thought prompting** since it provides an example. The version of Chain-of-thought prompting that is Zero-shot would not provide examples, but simply tell the LLM to break down the answer 'step by step'. The reason Chain-of-thought prompting is important is because LLMs often have trouble with math, or complex reasoning, but performs much better when it explicitly lists the intermediate steps.

There is much more that could be covered on this topic, but we will close out this section with a word on the timing of the prompt and how this can be used to help make Gen AI safe, and reliable. Many developers use prompts at different levels to provide better results. For example, the prompt the user inputs into the chat could then be delivered to the LLM with a system prompt asking it if this is a safe prompt. Here the system prompt will get a designation, and then decides what the system is to do with the prompts to ensure the prompt is safe, equitable, and appropriate [25]. If the prompt is determined to be acceptable, the output can then be generated only to be assessed again for appropriateness. A second system prompt could help the LLM evaluate the response to determine if the response breaks any guard rails the application developer may have put in place. Finally, once the response is determined appropriate, it can be returned to the user. This kind of prompt engineering pre-response, and post response are examples of how human prompts and system prompts work together to provide the best output possible.

Knowledge Bases

Knowledge bases are an important aspect of Generative AI for healthcare. One of the biggest challenges of Gen AI is the complication of hallucinations; or to use a medical term, confabulation. The answers are wrong but often have a ring of truth, which is one of the dangers of Gen AI. Knowledge bases are one of the tools developers use to limit hallucinations. A knowledge base can be any collection of data that the model is constrained to use when answering questions or following prompt instructions [26]. For example, you can place medical records for your patient panel in a storage, or database, and point the LLM to those as the definitive data sources for all questions or tasks asked of the LLM. If the LLM cannot derive the answer from the assigned data sources, then it returns an answer that it cannot provide the answer as requested.

Agents

Agents are another tool in the developer's toolbox that can help mitigate the limitations of LLMs [27]. Think of agents as computer assistants that help organize the use of the LLM to achieve a goal. Let us use a clinical example for primary care physicians, and tie together a few concepts we have already discussed.

The ACME Health Informatics staff built an application that uses agents to automatically collect the preventive medicine and health maintenance data for patients to be seen each day by every primary care clinician at the ACME ambulatory clinic. They assign an agent to collect the lipid profile, calculate the 10-year Framingham Risk score, and then use the data to evaluate the next steps for each patient by interrogating a knowledge base of the most recent ACC/AHA cholesterol guidelines. These results are sent to providers at the beginning of every day, so they are armed with information on their patients. There could also be an agent for breast cancer screening, colorectal cancer screening, and on and on.

Naturally, it would be important to realize these are only recommendations as it can often be the case that there are nuances to the individual's patient care that will affect the actual management. It could be intolerance or allergies to medications, patient preference, or a multitude of other reasons. The end user should also understand that the Informatics team would have performed many tests to validate the results to ensure the application is not introducing risk.

Retrieval Augmented Generation (RAG)

This is a very popular method used to minimize hallucinations [28]. RAG describes the process that takes place when the LLM is limited to just the information available in the knowledge base or repository of information the LLM has access to. This is also a way to customize a general model and train it for specific use cases as we mentioned in the earlier example about the cholesterol recommendation app. In that example, the app used both a knowledge base of the cholesterol guidelines and a database with the patient's clinical data.

How does RAG work? There are two parts to a RAG system: the retrieval system and the LLM. As mentioned above, the retrieval system reaches out to a data source to answer the question or task the user has input into the system. It does this by matching the numerical vectors, embeddings, of the prompt with the numerical vectors, embeddings, of the knowledge base. When the knowledge base is created, an embeddings model divides the knowledge base into chunks of information that it then converts into embeddings. These embeddings are used to determine the appropriate response to the prompt, and when selected will be added to the prompt and sent to the LLM for interpretation. The LLM takes the augmented prompt and produces a response to the user [29].

Benefits & Limitations

In the light of the heavy administrative burden of clinicians, it is easy to see the appeal of Gen AI. The efficiency that using Gen AI would potentially bring to this aspect of clinical work could significantly improve the quality of life for medical personnel. However, there are many use cases for Gen AI (See Chap. 6). Below is a limited list of examples:

Clinical Documentation

- AI-Powered Ambient Scribe
- Prior Authorization & Justification of Treatment Decision for Insurance
- Writing the First Draft of Discharge Summaries
- Evaluating Medication Reconciliation to reduce Medication Errors
- Summary letters from Specialist to Primary Care

Education and Learning

- Alternative Paths for Medical Education via Role Playing
- Gamification of Interaction with Virtual Patients
- Generation of Case Scenarios and Quizzes to Enhance Knowledge through Practice

Patient Engagement

- Virtual Assistants
- Personalized Learning & Question Answering

Research

- Coding for Analysis
- Text and Data Management
- Literature Summarization
- Drug Discovery
- Clinical Trials

These potential uses depend greatly on the accuracy of the output from Gen AI, which brings to the fore the concerns of using Gen AI in healthcare. The big issues are privacy, safety, misuse, misinformation, and bias. These can lead to lack of trust by users, and are critical issues to address before Gen AI can be used meaningfully in healthcare.

Though hallucinations have been mentioned several times previously, we need to return to this topic to discuss the dangers of this output in healthcare. One of the key factors that can contribute to this challenge is training data. After Google obtained Reddit data as mentioned earlier in this chapter, they rolled out their Artificial Intelligence Search feature which reportedly told some users that using "non-toxic glue" would help make cheese stick to pizza better [30]. In another example, the search engine responded that geologists recommend humans eat one rock per day [31]. These mistakes made the news cycle, and are not really in danger of being taken seriously, but they are shining examples of how questionable data can affect the output. In healthcare, these silly examples could turn serious if they provide misinformation about drugs, vaccines, or other interventions that could endanger the life of a patient. You will read in Chap. 13 of this textbook about the cybersecurity risks associated with LLMs, which is why data should be deidentified to minimize risk of privacy violations.

Additionally, there will be other areas that discuss ethical considerations in terms of avoiding inequities and bias. All of which are profoundly important. But I want to return to something we mentioned in the fundamentals of AI chapter: explainability. Plain and simple—there needs to be explainability when using AI in healthcare. This means there needs to be humans in the loop, where validation and assurances are prioritized to make AI safe to use in healthcare. We need to explore governance models, such as the Governance Model for AI in Healthcare, to ensure there is fairness, transparency, trustworthiness, and accountability [32].

Conclusion

Generative AI is an exciting new development that holds great promise for helping clinicians and patients navigate through the healthcare world. Furthermore, this area will develop at a rapid pace, which will make keeping track of this technology challenging, but it is important to approach development of these tools with care due to the high risks associated with implementing new technology for healthcare delivery by establishing a structured governance model to ensure AI is used responsibly, and safely.

Limitations and Challenges of AI

In the daily practice of medicine, risk and benefits are evaluated, or should be, with each intervention decision made. I would posit AI should be no different. However, this will take intentionality by clinicians and by regulatory agencies as many times AI can be embedded into systems that abstract away its reliance from the clinician.

So what are the risks of using AI? Here we'll share a list of considerations but it should not be considered all encompassing because it is certainly possible new ones will arise in the future.

One of the biggest risks in healthcare has always been data security and privacy as acknowledged by the enactment of the Health Insurance Portability and Accountability Act in 1996. Back then, it was all about managing paper records, but today it is an even bigger challenge with the ease of portability of electronic records. The risk is compounded by the use of the patient's records to train models if the models are not sufficiently secured. There have been numerous instances where bad actors have stolen records from healthcare systems, and this will be a challenge with future AI models, especially language models, if not addressed.

As mentioned in the previous chapter, another challenge with AI was uncovered in 1997 when Cooper et al. performed a study using machine learning to predict mortality in patients with pneumonia [33]. The goal was to provide a model that could predict the patients who had a high probability of death. This could help ambulatory clinicians admit the high risk patients to reduce mortality from pneumonia. They used a neural net to evaluate the data and found that the neural net outperformed the logistic regression model by a large margin (AUC 0.86 versus 0.77). The only problem was that when they looked at the data and the rules the neural net created from the data—they noted that the neural net predicted patients with asthma had a lower risk of mortality. As they dug into the data used by the neural net for training, they realized that the patients with asthma were actually hospitalized more often than non asthmatics in favor of aggressive treatment, and as a result had a lower mortality than the non asthmatic group. This highlighted the need to explainability of the results when using AI, which led to them championing the concept of intelligible machine learning models.

Unfortunately, mistakes, and bad outcomes, are part of medicine. And though no one ever wants harm to come to a patient, it still happens. The question is rarely who is responsible. That question is usually very clear from the medical record of who provided the care for the patient. However, what if the mistake occurred as a result of what an AI model recommended? What if the clinician dutifully executed the recommendation made by the system and that recommendation was flawed? Who is responsible? The clinician or the system that led the clinician astray? These are the future issues healthcare will need to address before there is wide implementation of AI systems.

Finally, we could talk about the ethics of using AI that has not been proven (in other words experimental), the lack of consent to use patient data for training AI models, the risk of disparities in care based on biased training data used by AI systems, and much, much more. The important thread that weaves through all these issues that the healthcare community needs to be involved and engaged to ensure we champion the use of AI that is responsible, ethical, and humane. We need to be the bridge between the technical advancements and the implementation in our practices.

References

1. Levi D. ChatGPT crosses 1 million users five days after launch. Tech Startups. Published December 5, 2022. Available at: https://techstartups.com. Accessed 5 Oct 2024.
2. NVIDIA. Efficiently scale LLM training across a large GPU cluster with Alpa and Ray. NVIDIA Developer Blog. Available at: https://developer.nvidia.com. Accessed 5 Oct 2024.
3. TrendForce. GPU demand from ChatGPT could reach 30,000 chips as it readies for commercialization. TrendForce. Published March 1, 2023. Available at: https://www.trendforce.com. Accessed 5 Oct 2024.
4. Zuckerberg M. Meta Is Buying 350,000 Nvidia H100 GPUs for AGI. The Register. Published January 20, 2024. Available at: https://www.theregister.com. Accessed 5 Oct 2024.
5. The Independent. Reddit strikes $60 million deal allowing Google to train AI models on its posts. Published February 22, 2024. Available at: https://www.independent.co.uk. Accessed 5 Oct 2024.
6. Arize AI. Breaking down Meta's Llama 3 herd of models. Available at: https://arize.com. Accessed 5 Oct 2024.
7. Common Crawl. Overview. Available at: https://commoncrawl.org/overview. Accessed 5 Oct 2024.
8. The Pile. Available at: https://pile.eleuther.ai/. Accessed 5 Oct 2024.
9. NVIDIA. Generative AI. NVIDIA. https://www.nvidia.com/en-us/glossary/generative-ai/. Accessed 6 Oct 2024.
10. IBM Developer. Token optimization: the backbone of effective prompt engineering. Available at: https://developer.ibm.com/articles/awb-token-optimization-backbone-of-effective-prompt-engineering. Accessed 5 Oct 2024.
11. Vaswani A, Shazeer N, Parmar N, Uszkoreit J, Jones L, Gomez AN, et al. Attention is all you need, Adv Neural Inf Process Syst. 2017;30:5998–6008.
12. Dang V, Bendersky M, Croft WB. An overview on Large Language Models. SpringerLink; 2023. Available at: https://link.springer.com. Accessed 5 Oct 2024.
13. Vellum AI. Comparing Llama 3.170b vs GPT-4o mini vs. Gemini 1.5 Flash vs. Claude 3.5 Haiku on three tasks. Vellum AI Blog. https://www.vellum.ai/blog/llama-3-1-70b-vs-gpt-4o-vs-claude-3-5-sonnet. Accessed 6 Oct 2024.
14. Turing. The necessity of bias in neural networks. Turing Knowledge Base. https://www.turing.com/kb/necessity-of-bias-in-neural-networks. Accessed 6 Oct 2024.
15. IBM. LLM benchmarks. IBM. https://www.ibm.com/think/topics/llm-benchmarks. Published 2024. Accessed 6 Oct 2024.
16. Anthropic. Claude 3.5 Sonnet model types. Anthropic. https://www.anthropic.com/news/claude-3-5-sonnet. Published 2024. Accessed 6 Oct 2024.
17. Huang K, Altosaar J, Ranganath R. ClinicalBERT: Modeling clinical notes and predicting hospital readmission. arXiv. https://arxiv.org/abs/1904.05342. Published 2019. Accessed 6 Oct 2024.
18. Gu Y, Tinn R, Cheng H, Lucas M, Usuyama N, Liu X, et al. Domain-specific language model pretraining for biomedical natural language processing. ACM Trans Comput Biol Bioinform. 2021;19(3):1–14. https://doi.org/10.1145/3458754.
19. Li Y, Rao S, Solares RA, Hassaine A, Ramakrishnan R, Canoy D, et al. BEHRT: transformer for electronic health records. Sci Rep. 2020;10(1):7155. https://doi.org/10.1038/s41598-020-62922-y.

20. Luo R, Sun L, Xia Y, Qin T, Zhang S, Poon H, et al. BioGPT: generative pre-trained transformer for biomedical text generation and mining. Brief Bioinform. 2023;24(1):bbac409.
21. Abbas A, Rehman MS, Rehman SS. Comparing the performance of Popular large language models on the national board of medical examiners sample questions. Cureus. 2024;16(3):e55991.
22. Singhal K, Azizi S, Tu T, Mahdavi SS, Wei J, Chung HW, et al. Large language models encode clinical knowledge. Nature. 2023;620:172–80.
23. Singhal K, Azizi S, Tu T, et al. Towards expert-level medical question answering with large language models. arXiv. https://arxiv.org/pdf/2305.09617. Published May 2023. Accessed 6 Oct 2024.
24. OpenAI. Optimizing LLMs for accuracy. OpenAI Platform. https://platform.openai.com/docs/guides/optimizing-llm-accuracy. Accessed 6 Oct 2024.
25. Zheng Z, Liu Y, Chen H, et al. On prompt-driven safeguarding for large language models. arXiv. arXiv:2401.18018v2 [cs.LG]. Published March 4, 2024. Accessed at https://arxiv.org/html/2401.18018v26 on 6 Oct 2024.
26. Chen X, Liu C, Huang H, et al. Reducing hallucinations in large language models through knowledge base integration. J Artif Intell Res. 2023;78:567–90.
27. Johnson M, Gupta A, Patel R, et al. Enhancing large language models with autonomous agents for improved task performance and reliability. IEEE Trans Neural Netw Learn Syst. 2023;34(8):3456–68.
28. Lewis P, Karpukhin V, Oguz B, et al. Retrieval-augmented generation for knowledge-intensive NLP tasks. Adv Neural Inf Process Syst. 2020;33:9459–74.
29. Yogatama D, Han X, Borgeaud S, et al. Retrieval-augmented generation: combining retrieval and generative models for effective knowledge-intensive tasks. arXiv. https://arxiv.org/abs/2107.07566. Published July 2021. Accessed 6 Oct 2024.
30. Kelly J. Google AI suggests glue for pizza: viral blunders highlight challenges in AI search. Forbes. https://www.forbes.com/sites/jackkelly/2024/05/31/google-ai-glue-to-pizza-viral-blunders/. Published May 31, 2024. Accessed 6 Oct 2024.
31. Glue pizza and eat rocks: Google AI search errors go viral. BBC News. https://www.bbc.com/news/articles/cd11gzejgz4o. Published May 26, 2024. Accessed 6 Oct 2024.
32. Reddy S. Evaluating large language models for use in healthcare: a framework for translational value assessment. Informatics Med Unlocked. 2023;41:101304.
33. Cooper GF, Aliferis CF, Ambrosino R, et al. An evaluation of machine-learning methods for predicting pneumonia mortality. Artif Intell Med. 1997;9(2):107–38.

Part II
AI Use Cases in Clinical Care, Administration and Research

Chapter 6
Current and Emerging Uses of Generative AI for Clinical Care, Administration, and Research

Terry Adirim

Introduction

AI is rapidly transforming various business sectors by enhancing efficiency, accuracy, and innovation. AI is utilized commonly in retail and e-commerce, manufacturing, transportation, and telecommunications industries, including being used prominently for marketing and advertising, logistics, and human resources. One of the most prominent sectors where AI is being heavily utilized is the financial industry where AI is employed for tasks such as fraud detection, algorithmic trading, and customer service automation. Other uses include customer service bots and virtual assistants in banking and insurance that provide instant responses to customer inquiries, improving service quality and operational efficiency [1].

The healthcare sector can learn from the AI experiences in other industries to benefit healthcare delivery and administration. Generative AI (Gen AI) presents a wide array of potential applications in clinical care most especially for completing repetitive administrative tasks and in supporting research. The difference between healthcare and other industries is healthcare's unique privacy and regulatory requirements and concerns for patient safety of new technology. Therefore, the clinician must be cognizant of these concerns when adopting these AI powered tools.

It is expected that Gen AI will significantly impact diagnostics, treatment, and patient management. Additionally, Gen AI has the potential to streamline and enhance various administrative tasks in healthcare, leading to increased efficiency, reduced costs, and improved accuracy. This chapter will cover current and potential use cases for AI in healthcare, uses that are rapidly evolving with new innovations and therefore does not provide an exhaustive list.

T. Adirim (✉)
Departments of Pediatrics and Preventive Medicine and Biostatistics,
Uniformed Services University of the Health Sciences, Bethesda, MD, USA

T. Adirim (ed.), *Digital Health, AI and Generative AI in Healthcare*,
https://doi.org/10.1007/978-3-031-83526-1_6

AI Uses to Support Clinical Work

Diagnostics

Artificial Intelligence (AI) in clinical diagnostics has the potential to transform how diseases are detected, diagnosed, and monitored by leveraging machine learning (ML), deep learning, and natural language processing (NLP) to analyze large and complex datasets. AI-powered diagnostic tools have shown remarkable capabilities in interpreting medical images, analyzing genetic data, and predicting patient outcomes, leading to earlier detection of diseases, more accurate diagnoses, and improved patient care [2].

One of the most commonly used applications of AI for clinical diagnosis is medical imaging. AI algorithms, particularly those based on deep learning, have demonstrated exceptional accuracy in interpreting radiological images, often matching or even surpassing human experts in specific tasks. AI enhances MRI, CT, and X-ray images to improve clarity and aid in the detection of abnormalities. For example, Google's DeepMind developed an AI system capable of analyzing retinal scans to detect over 50 eye conditions, such as diabetic retinopathy and age-related macular degeneration, with accuracy comparable to that of expert ophthalmologists [3]. Similarly, the AI system **CheXNet** was designed to detect pneumonia from chest X-rays. Trained on a large dataset of over 100,000 images, CheXNet can identify pneumonia with a sensitivity higher than radiologists, which is critical for early diagnosis and treatment [4]. Moreover, AI is being used to generate synthetic images to augment training datasets for radiologists [5].

AI is also revolutionizing the field of pathology by supporting the generation of high-resolution images of tissue samples for more accurate diagnosis of diseases like cancer [6]. Another use case in pathology includes simulating various disease states to train pathologists.

AI in the field of Dermatology is supporting education and diagnoses by creating synthetic images of skin conditions to improve diagnostic algorithms. Also, AI is assisting in the diagnosis of skin diseases by generating comparisons with known conditions [7].

Treatment Planning

An exciting use of Gen AI is to support personalized medicine. AI has the potential to generate personalized treatment plans based on patient-specific data, including genetics, lifestyle, and medical history [1].

Another area for AI use is planning for radiation therapy. AI can design optimized radiation treatment plans by generating different scenarios and predicting outcomes [8]. Similarly, AI can be used for surgical planning by creating 3D models of patient anatomy to assist surgeons in planning complex procedures. Additionally, AI can generate simulations of surgical procedures to improve surgical techniques and outcomes [9, 10].

Patient Monitoring and Management

Since the pandemic, remote patient monitoring (RPM) has accelerated in use. AI can support RPM by generating alerts and insights from continuous patient data streams (e.g., from wearables) to detect early signs of complications [11].

Another area AI can be useful is in supporting chronic disease management. AI has the potential to create personalized care plans for managing chronic diseases like diabetes and hypertension, including proposing patient tailored diet, exercise, and medication schedules. AI-powered virtual health assistants have the potential to help patients by providing real-time advice and reminders to patients based on their health data and treatment plans.

Clinical Decision Support and Precision Medicine

Physicians are familiar with clinical algorithms that serve as clinical support tools. Often, they are integrated into electronic health records systems. These algorithms are often developed by specialty society committees for treatment of patient medical conditions and tend to be static requiring updating as new evidence emerges [12]. Generative AI has the potential to facilitate real time or near real time updating based on changes in the medical literature and expert recommendations.

Another useful area for clinical decision support is for managing drug interactions and prediction of side effects based on patient specific data [13]. Also, Gen AI has the potential to be used to predict treatment outcomes by creating models that use patient specific data including medical history, lab and radiological results and genetic data, that can predict the likely outcomes of different treatment options to support physician decision-making.

Patient Communication and Documentation

Patient communication is an area being explored to improve patient outcomes and experience. Tools under development and being piloted have the potential to improve patient health literacy and experience and include AI tools for generating automated reports and care summaries of office and hospital visits and for creating personalized patient education materials [14]. One of the most exciting use cases for AI is ambient dictation, that uses AI to record and in real time transcribe conversations between patients and clinicians that is automatically added to the patients electronic health record. This technology has the potential to improve the quality of the patient physician encounter and reduce administrative burden (see below for more details).

Emergency Care

One area that is being explored to support emergency departments is AI supported Triage. Triage is an important first step for patients entering emergency care to determine priority of care. Triage is algorithm based, and generative AI can be deployed to generate more precise algorithms and risk stratification and has the potential to customize triage scores based on patient specific history using EHR data [15, 16].

Rehabilitation and Therapy

AI has the potential to support clinical decision making, outcome prediction and augment patient engagement for rehabilitation programs, specifically creating personalized rehabilitation programs for patients recovering from surgery or injury [17].

Another promising area is use of AI to facilitate and expand access to mental health therapy. With a national shortage of mental health care providers AI can provide support by improving the time to identifying high risk individuals with mental health diagnoses to prioritize interventions Also, AI can support therapists by generating personalized therapy plans and virtual companions to support mental health treatment. AI might also have the potential to identify individuals at risk for developing mental health conditions so that preventative treatments can be given [18, 19].

Infection Control

Infection control can be enhanced through AI powered infection spread modeling techniques. AI can generate models to predict the spread of infections within healthcare settings and inform control measures [20]. Another potential use includes antimicrobial stewardship to facilitate the creation of guidelines for the use of antimicrobials to prevent resistance and optimize treatment. Clinicians are often confronted with antibiotic treatment decisions prior to available culture data and so choose broad spectrum drugs that increases the risk of antibiotic resistance. AI has the potential to provide individualized recommendations for narrower spectrum options based on a patient's history and resistance patterns within the community [21].

Generative AI to Reduce Administrative Burden

Documentation and Reporting

AI powered ambient dictation technology (also known as ambient scribes) has the potential to revolutionize clinician documentation by integrating into clinical workflows and capturing patient encounters in real-time. This technology leverages advanced natural language processing (NLP) and speech recognition algorithms to transcribe spoken interactions between clinicians and patients into structured electronic health record (EHR) entries. By reducing the administrative burden of transcribing encounters in real time, ambient dictation allows clinicians to focus more on the patient and less on manual data entry, thereby potentially improving efficiency and reducing burnout. Moreover, it can enhance the accuracy and completeness of medical records, contributing to better patient outcomes and streamlined healthcare operations. However, studies have been mixed with some showing that AI powered ambient dictation can significantly decrease the time spent on documentation, leading to more effective and satisfactory clinical practice while some recent studies have shown little difference in clinician time in the EHR [22, 23]. Some studies including one of the largest to date have shown positive clinician experience with Ambient AI tools including reduced clinician cognitive burden, workload and burnout [24–26]. While ambient AI documentation has been found to be acceptable to physicians and patients, caution is important because these tools can produce discrepancies and introduce potential errors that require the clinician to review and edit to ensure accuracy [22]. Other documentation use cases include generating discharge summaries and subspecialty consultations that can be augmented with AI by utilizing data in a patients EHR to automatically generate these reports upon demand [27]. Note that introducing any of these new tools into the clinician workflow requires training and support for successful adoption and monitoring of its use to ensure quality and patient safety.

Another area of documentation where AI can reduce burden on providers is medical coding and billing. AI tools are being developed to automatically generate medical codes (e.g., ICD-10, CPT) from clinical documentation and to create accurate and compliant billing statements and claims. There are emerging tools being piloted at large medical centers, but these tools are not yet commonly deployed [28].

Just as AI is supporting automation of medical coding, medical administrative start-ups are creating tools to automate the entire process involved in revenue cycle management and claims processing, administrative functions that are complex and heavily regulated. AI can generate detailed financial reports, including revenue, expenses, and profit margins. Also, like for other industries, AI can support quicker and automated tracking of accounts receivable and accounts payable. This can be tied to claims processing by creating and submitting insurance claims with accurate coding and documentation. And lastly, providers can automate the follow-up and resolution of denied or delayed claims.

Another administrative burden that AI can address includes regulatory compliance reporting automatically generating reports, for Centers for Medicare and Medicaid Services (CMS) programs that require reporting of quality metrics and adherence to healthcare standards. CMS requires providers, hospitals, ambulatory centers, physicians, to report on hundreds of measures to ensure compliance with performance standards and improve patient care. AI can facilitate the electronic reporting of these measures by automating extraction of data from EHRs and other health IT systems.

Patient Scheduling and Management

Appointment Scheduling is another administrative burden on practices that can be supported and automated by AI. Managing appointments can be frustrating and takes up administrative personnel's time. Moreover, managing patient "no-shows" can also be frustrating. AI can generate optimal schedules for patient appointments, reducing conflicts and no-shows.

Another potential use for AI is patient intake and registration. AI can support the creation of patient specific digital forms for intake and registration, for generating patient profiles for the visit and updating electronic health records (EHRs).

An interesting area includes automated responses to common patient inquiries via chatbots. This application in AI is being piloted in some places and it's not known whether these will be accepted by patients who may prefer direct interaction with a physician or other clinician [29].

Practice and Hospital Operations Management

AI is particularly effective for repetitive tasks and support of operations. AI tools can automate the generation of analytical reports on hospital performance, patient outcomes, and operational efficiency. Also, AI can support creating dashboards and visualizations in real time to support data-driven decision-making.

Another operations requirement that AI can support includes resource allocation decisions. AI can generate schedules for staff shifts and optimize the allocation of medical personnel. Also, AI can automate the management of hospital resources like rooms, equipment, and ensure precise supply chain management through the generation of inventory reports, forecasting supply needs, automating procurement processes, and managing vendor relationships.

Other administrative processes where AI is currently being used are for personnel management including recruitment and onboarding of new personnel. Like other industries, healthcare providers can generate job descriptions, postings, and candidate performance evaluation reports.

Other healthcare business use cases that AI can support and improve are legal compliance, customer service, marketing and community outreach.

Other Use Cases for AI

Drug Development and Clinical Trials

Artificial Intelligence (AI) in drug development and clinical trials is transforming how new pharmaceuticals are discovered, tested, and brought to market. AI technologies, including machine learning (ML), deep learning, and natural language processing (NLP), have been instrumental in accelerating various stages of drug development. By rapidly analyzing vast datasets, predicting molecular interactions, and even identifying potential drug candidates, AI reduces the time and cost traditionally associated with bringing new drugs to market.

One of the primary applications of AI in drug discovery is in virtual screening and drug design. AI algorithms can screen millions of chemical compounds to predict which are most likely to bind to a target protein associated with a disease. This process dramatically shortens the drug discovery timeline, which often involves years of laboratory research. For example, the British AI company Exscientia, in collaboration with Sumitomo Dainippon Pharma, used AI to develop a drug for obsessive-compulsive disorder (OCD) named DSP-1181 [30]. This drug candidate was identified in less than 12 months, compared to the typical 4–5 years using traditional methods. AI-driven platforms like Exscientia's enable the rapid design and optimization of drug candidates by predicting their pharmacological properties, efficacy, and safety profiles.

AI also plays a significant role in repurposing existing drugs for new therapeutic indications. Drug repurposing can be highly efficient, as it involves compounds that have already been tested for safety in humans, bypassing early stages of clinical trials. BenevolentAI used its AI-based platform to analyze vast amounts of biomedical data and identified baricitinib, an existing drug used for rheumatoid arthritis, as a potential treatment for COVID-19 [31]. This discovery led to clinical trials and the subsequent emergency use authorization of baricitinib for treating severe COVID-19 cases. The ability of AI to analyze complex biological data and suggest new therapeutic uses for existing drugs highlights its potential to quickly address emerging health crises.

In clinical trials, AI aids in patient recruitment and trial design. Recruiting eligible patients for clinical trials is often a slow and challenging process, but AI can streamline this by sifting through electronic health records (EHRs) to identify suitable candidates based on factors such as genetic profiles, demographics, and medical histories. For instance, IBM Watson Health has developed AI algorithms that help match patients to clinical trials more accurately, thus speeding up the recruitment process and increasing the likelihood of trial success [32]. AI also assists in monitoring patient responses during trials by analyzing data from wearable devices and other health monitoring systems, providing real-time insights into the drug's effects and safety.

Additionally, AI can facilitate predictive modeling of drug responses, aiding in the identification of biomarkers for patient stratification. Machine learning techniques are used to construct causal models that can predict how patients will respond to specific therapies [33]. This technology enables the development of personalized treatment regimens, which can significantly enhance the efficacy of drugs while minimizing adverse effects. By predicting patient responses, AI-driven models contribute to more targeted and efficient clinical trials, potentially leading to faster regulatory approvals.

However, despite the clear potential of AI in drug development, challenges remain. AI models require high-quality, diverse datasets to function effectively, and data privacy concerns can limit access to such data. Additionally, the interpretability of AI algorithms is crucial, especially for regulatory submissions where understanding the decision-making process behind AI-driven predictions is necessary [34]. Nonetheless, with the growing success of AI applications, pharmaceutical companies and research institutions continue to explore and expand their role in making drug development more efficient, precise, and cost-effective.

References

1. Bharadiya J, Thomas R, Ahmed F. Rise of artificial intelligence in business and industry. J Eng Res Rep. 2023;25:100807.
2. Yu KH, Beam AL, Kohane IS. Artificial intelligence in healthcare. Nat Biomed Eng. 2018;2(10):719–31.
3. De Fauw J, Ledsam JR, Romera-Paredes B, Nikolov S, Tomasev N, Blackwell S, et al. Clinically applicable deep learning for diagnosis and referral in retinal disease. Nat Med. 2018;24(9):1342–50.
4. Raipukar P, Irvin J, Zhu K, et al. CheXNet: Radiologist-level pneumonia detection on chest X-rays with deep learning. arXiv. 2017;1711.05225v3. Published December 25, 2017. https://arxiv.org/abs/1711.05225. Accessed 7 Oct 2024.
5. Kitsios F, Kamariotou M, Syngelakis AI, Talias MA. Recent advances of artificial intelligence in healthcare: a systematic literature review. Appl Sci. 2023;13(13):7479. https://doi.org/10.3390/app13137479.
6. Chang J, Hatfield B. Advancements in computer vision and pathology: unraveling the potential of artificial intelligence for precision diagnosis and beyond. Adv Cancer Res. 2024;161:431–78.
7. Clark Lambert W, Grzybowski A. Dermatology and artificial intelligence. Clin Dermatol. 2024;42(3):207–9.
8. Pillai M, Adapa K, Das SK, Mazur L, Dooley J, Marks LB, et al. Using artificial intelligence to improve the quality and safety of radiation therapy. J Am Coll Radiol. 2019;16(9 Pt B):1267–72.
9. Mangano FG, Admakin O, Lerner H, Mangano C. Artificial intelligence and augmented reality for guided implant surgery planning: a proof of concept. J Dent. 2023;133:104485.
10. Ghaednia H, Fourman MS, Lans A, Detels K, Dijkstra H, Lloyd S, et al. Augmented and virtual reality in spine surgery, current applications and future potentials. Spine J. 2021;21(10):1617–25.

11. Palanisamy P, Padmanabhan A, Ramasamy A, Subramaniam S. Remote patient activity monitoring system by integrating IoT sensors and artificial intelligence techniques. Sensors (Basel). 2023;23(13):5869. Published 2023 Jun 25.
12. Magrabi F, Ammenwerth E, McNair JB, De Keizer NF, Hyppönen H, Nykänen P, et al. Artificial intelligence in clinical decision support: challenges for evaluating AI and practical implications. Yearb Med Inform. 2019;28(1):128–34.
13. Zhang Y, Deng Z, Xu X, Feng Y, Junliang S. Application of artificial intelligence in drug-drug interactions prediction: a review. J Chem Inf Model. 2024;64(7):2158–73.
14. Tse G, Kuzma N, Khan A. Perspective: artificial intelligence and patient communication. J Hosp Med. https://doi.org/10.1002/jhm.13301. Published online February 10, 2024.
15. Karlafti E, Anagnostis A, Simou T, Kollatou AS, Paramythiotis D, Kaiafa G, et al. Support systems of clinical decisions in the triage of the emergency department using artificial intelligence: the efficiency to support triage. Acta Med Litu. 2023;30(1):19–25.
16. Farahmand S, Shabestari O, Pakrah M, Hossein-Nejad H, Arbab M, Bagheri-Hariri S. Artificial intelligence-based triage for patients with acute abdominal pain in emergency department; a diagnostic accuracy study. Adv J Emerg Med. 2017;1(1):e5. Published 2017 Oct 21.
17. Tack C. Artificial intelligence and machine learning | applications in musculoskeletal physiotherapy. Musculoskelet Sci Pract. 2019;39:164–9.
18. Lee EE, Torous J, De Choudhury M, Depp CA, Graham SA, Kim HC, et al. Artificial intelligence for mental health care: clinical applications, barriers, facilitators, and artificial wisdom. Biol Psychiatry Cogn Neurosci Neuroimaging. 2021;6(9):856–64.
19. Pham KT, Nabizadeh A, Selek S. Artificial intelligence and chatbots in psychiatry. Psychiatry Q. 2022;93(1):249–53.
20. Qi ZY, Zhao PY, Geng SH, Yi HM, Yang LP. COVID-19 Epidemic: possibility of Artificial Intelligence in Infection Control and Prevention. J Epidemiol. 2020;30(8):371. https://doi.org/10.2188/jea.JE20200203. Epub 2020 Jun 6.
21. Chang A, Chen JH. BSAC Vanguard Series: artificial intelligence and antibiotic stewardship. J Antimicrob Chemother. 2022;77(5):1216–7.
22. Tierney AA, Gayre G, Hoberman B, Mattern B, Ballesca M, Kipnis P, et al. Ambient artificial intelligence scribes to alleviate the burden of clinical documentation. NEJM Catal Innov Care Deliv. 2024;5(3). https://doi.org/10.1056/CAT.23.0404.
23. Balloch J, Sridharan S, Oldham G, Wray J, Gough P, Robinson R, et al. Use of an ambient artificial intelligence tool to improve quality of clinical documentation. Future Healthc J. 2024;11(3):100157. Published 2024 Jun 26.
24. MIsurac J, Knake LA, Blum JM. The effect of Ambient artificial intelligence notes on provider burnout. Appl Clin Inform. https://doi.org/10.1055/a-2461-4576. Published online November 5, 2024.
25. Owens LM, Wilda JJ, Hahn PY, Koehler T, Fletcher JJ. The association between use of ambient voice technology documentation during primary care patient encounters, documentation burden, and provider burnout. Fam Pract. 2024;41(2):86–91.
26. Tierney AA, Gayre G, Hoberman B, et al. Ambient artificial intelligence scribes: learnings after 1 year and over 2.5 million uses. NEJM Catalyst Innov Care Deliv. 2025;6(5). Published online March 31, 2025.
27. Kachman MM, Brennan I, Oskvarek JJ, Waseem T, Pines JM. How artificial intelligence could transform emergency care. Am J Emerg Med. 2024;81:40–6.
28. Siwicki B. How AI is transforming medical coding for physicians and coders. Healthcare IT News. https://www.healthcareitnews.com/news/how-ai-transforming-medical-coding-physicians-and-coders. Published March 21, 2023. Accessed 9 Aug 2024.
29. Ayers JW, Poliak A, Dredze M, Leas EC, Zhu Z, Kelley JB, et al. Comparing physician and artificial intelligence chatbot responses to patient questions posted to a public social media forum. JAMA Intern Med. 2023;183(6):589–96.
30. Wills T. AI drug discovery: assessing the first AI-designed drug candidates to go into human clinical trials. American Chemical Society. September 23, 2022. https://www.cas.org/resources/cas-insights/ai-drug-discovery-assessing-the-first-ai-designed-drug-candidates-to-go-into-human-clinical-trials. Accessed 20 Nov 2024.

31. Richardson PJ, Robinson BWS, Smith DP, Stebbing J. The AI-assisted identification and clinical efficacy of Baricitinib in the treatment of COVID-19. Vaccines (Basel). 2022;10(6):951. Published 2022 Jun 15.
32. Piccialli F, di Cola VS, Giampaolo F, Cuomo S. The role of artificial intelligence in fighting the COVID-19 pandemic. Inf Syst Front. 2021;23(6):1467–97.
33. Kline A, Wang H, Li Y, Dennis S, Hutch M, Xu Z, et al. Multimodal machine learning in precision health: a scoping review. NPJ Digit Med. 2022;5:171.
34. Mak KK, Pichika MR. Artificial intelligence in drug development: present status and future prospects. Drug Discov Today. 2019;24(3):773–80.

Chapter 7
Artificial Intelligence in Pediatric Healthcare: Clinical Applications

Amy Molten and Alyssa Abo

Introduction

Overview of AI in Pediatric Healthcare

Historically, advances in technology for adults far outpaced those in pediatrics and the trend continues with respect to AI [1]. Fewer medical devices and digital health technologies are being developed specifically for children. Likewise, AI-enabled research and development in pediatric medicine lags. This limits its potential impact on public health, worsens child healthcare disparities, risks inappropriate use of adult tools for pediatric populations, and stifles future innovations in pediatric care.

In healthcare, it is common practice to use the quintuple aim as the guiding light or north star. The quintuple aim focuses on enhancing patient care, improving population health, reducing costs, improving the well-being of the workforce, and advancing health equity [2]. Advancing pediatric technologies promotes each part of the quintuple aim. To accelerate the development of pediatric technologies, several initiatives are underway, including the FDA's Pediatric Device Consortia Grants program and dedicated pediatric accelerators focused on pediatric technologies to help bridge the gap between pediatric and adult technology development. This chapter aims to highlight the opportunity for careful, ethical, and thoughtful integration of AI into pediatric healthcare.

A. Molten
Department of Pediatrics, Tufts Medical Center, Boston, MA, USA

A. Abo (✉)
Impact1 at Stanford Mussallem Center for Biodesign, Stanford Medicine, Stanford, CA, USA

T. Adirim (ed.), *Digital Health, AI and Generative AI in Healthcare*,
https://doi.org/10.1007/978-3-031-83526-1_7

Consideration of AI in Pediatric Healthcare

Why is there a technology gap in pediatric care? The reason is complicated and multi-factorial. One of the explanations is that the pediatric market is smaller than that for adults, and thus technologies developed for children and their caregivers may not have the same ability to scale [3]. But the business angle may not always hold true and is only one part of a larger divide in the innovation ecosystem. Developing pediatric technologies can be challenging since children are in a continuous state of growth and change. Additionally, the adoption of new technology requires buy-in from families, schools, caregivers and the pediatric medical community that adds to the complexity for technology development [3]. Children are considered vulnerable members of society due to their range of cognitive and decisional abilities and dependence on adults for care, decision-making, and consent. This heightens the obligation of health and technology professionals to act in their best interest, with increased pressure to get it right and do no harm. Effective machine learning models trained in adult patients are not necessarily transferable to pediatric patients and require quality pediatric-specific data that is not always readily available. In fact, pediatric data may be more coveted because the medical community is more cautious around this vulnerable population and understands that any negative use of pediatric data could have long-term consequences.

Nevertheless, pediatric patients from birth through 18 years of age, could benefit from advances in health AI (Fig. 7.1). The range of potential mirrors that of adults, with opportunity for diagnostic and therapeutic breakthroughs, supporting young patients and caregivers along the full spectrum of physical and mental health needs while promoting wellness and prevention initiatives as children grow. Furthermore, AI-based systems improvement could transform the pediatric care delivery experience, with the ability to improve administrative workflows and decrease burden at a time when fewer physicians are going into pediatrics and shortages are inevitable, particularly in rural and lower-resource communities. Clinicians could benefit from AI's ability to augment medical decision-making and diagnostic capabilities while enhancing remote monitoring and virtual care capabilities.

Health decisions and interventions in infancy and childhood can impact lifetime and even future generation potential. So, it is incumbent on those developing new AI-driven technology to not leave the pediatric community behind. Rather, we need to develop creative ways to bring together pediatric data and use it in a way that is responsible and ethical so that advances in technology can benefit the pediatric population and society as a whole.

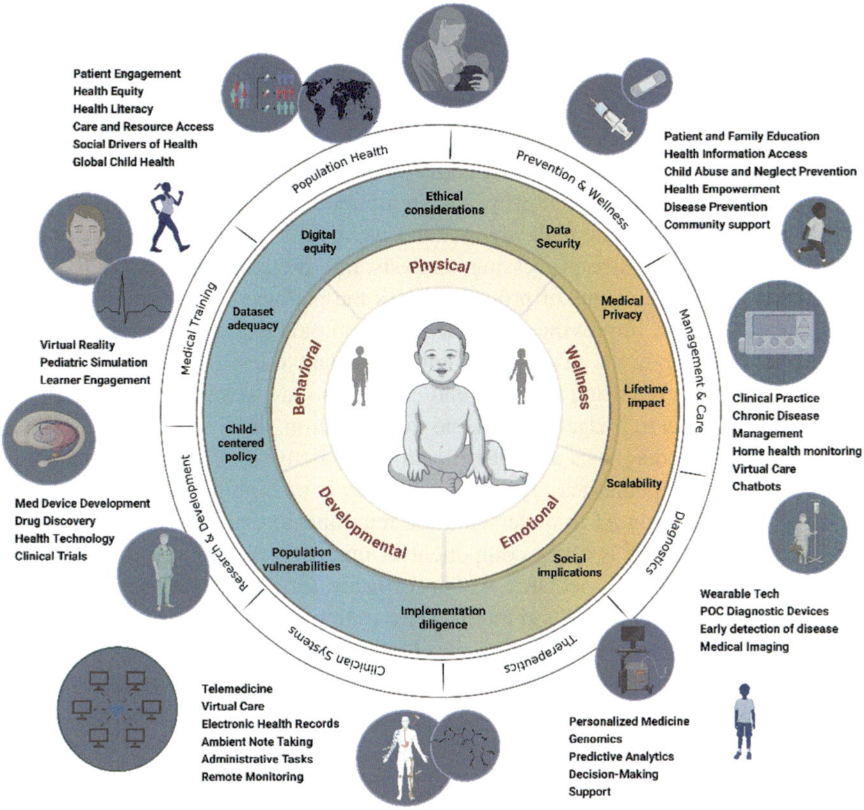

Fig. 7.1 Essential considerations for artificial intelligence in pediatric healthcare. This diagram highlights a number of key variables that should be integrated into research, development and implementation when artificial intelligence is applied to pediatric populations. Created with BioRender.com. (Permission to use by Dr. Amy Molten)

Clinical Practice

Medical Imaging

The incorporation of AI into diagnostics has been widespread, especially in medical imaging. AI has the potential to decrease time and costs associated with imaging as well as enhance interpretation. Unfortunately, despite the potential for AI in pediatric medical imaging, there has been limited advancement. According to the Data

Science Institute of the American College of Radiology (ACR), in 2023, only 3% of AI algorithms approved by the FDA were intended for pediatrics [4]. This AI gap for pediatrics is in part explained by limited pediatric datasets and the heterogeneity of the data as children grow [5]. Furthermore, there is a shortage of pediatric radiologists which could delay the development of AI algorithms. On the other hand, this creates an opportunity where AI could potentially help offset the gaps [6].

In the pediatric imaging pathway, AI can influence each part of the process from 'request to report.' [5] The pathway includes using AI from scheduling an appointment, to image acquisition processing, analysis, interpretation, and reporting. There have been some early signs of promise across the pathway and across the various imaging modalities. Improving image acquisition could decrease the time required for the study which in the case of MRI could translate to less time exposed to anesthesia for patients requiring sedation and could translate to lower radiation for CT scans. With respect to image analysis and interpretation, there is growing interest in AI algorithms for diagnosis and classification, predictive analytics, radiogenomics and biomarkers in pediatrics [5]. Radiogenomics is a combination of "radiomics" and "genomics" using AI to understand the relationship between medical imaging and genomic data and is a key component of precision medicine. Currently, software is being developed, pediatric AI consortia are forming, registries are growing to include pediatric patients, and multi-center initiatives are underway.

The technologies currently being developed cover a wide spectrum of disease states and are growing across imaging modalities. For example, there are a number of computer-based software algorithms to augment radiograph interpretation such as bone age determination, fracture detection, presence of pneumonia or developmental dysplasia of the hip [5]. CT technologies can be used to assess volume of pneumothoraces or degree of hydrocephalus and biomarkers were able to distinguish MRIs of patients with autism spectrum disorder from healthy patients [5]. The AI in the medical imaging market is expected to continue growing rapidly and be a $20B industry by 2030 and hopefully pediatrics will be a key area of growth [7].

Early Detection of Diseases

Another area of AI-guided diagnostic potential for pediatric patients is in the early detection of diseases. While our health needs and behaviors are patterned, individual patient barriers to ideal health are remarkably unique. This is especially true for infants and children. For this reason, pediatric medicine is necessarily transitioning from uniform approaches to diagnosis and treatment toward personalized, precision-based care. Considering each child's unique genetic, clinical, and environmental factors, this diagnostic revolution enables clinicians to diagnose and offer individualized medical therapies with remarkable speed, specificity, and efficacy.

For example, time to intervention is vitally important for a developing young brain, and when treating seriously ill children more broadly. So, consider the case described by Michelle Clark et al. of Rady Children's Institute for Genomic

Medicine [8]. A 3-day-old boy was admitted to the neonatal ICU with seizures and a strong family history of infantile seizures responsive to phenobarbital. The team's platform was built to analyze EHR data alongside genomic sequencing data from dried blood spots. Combining the rapid whole-genome sequencing method with automated AI-driven phenotyping and interpretation, rapid diagnosis of a pathogenic variant was made in just under 21 h. This was more than 27 h earlier than the diagnosis made concurrently with manual methods. In this case, the diagnosis provided confidence in treatment with phenobarbital and changed this child's prognosis.

This convergence of genomics and advanced computational analytics allows for the identification of patterns and relationships that may be too subtle or complex for traditional analysis methods to detect. Automated tools like these will become the new cornerstone of accurate rare genetic disease diagnosis, potentially refining traditional newborn screening techniques, and promoting life-saving changes to patient care.

Likewise, there is potential value in the application of AI for earlier diagnosis of more common pediatric conditions. For example, various studies have considered machine-learning-based early diagnosis of autism, either through analysis of eye movements or multimodular analysis of patient key behaviors combined with parent and clinician questionnaires [9–11]. Another study demonstrated that just five history encounters and a limited number of exposure variables were sufficient to predict BMI for both boys and girls in very early childhood [12]. Erika Chang et al. published a study showing that a machine learning model based on clinical features could effectively identify obstructive sleep apnea (OSA) in children, setting the stage for a potentially viable clinical alternative to nocturnal pediatric OSA [13]. And a novel machine learning model demonstrated the feasibility of differentiating between necrotizing enterocolitis and spontaneous intestinal perforation prior to intended surgical interventions, a critical time-sensitive distinction for many preterm neonates [14].

Another example of active diagnostic research is in the setting of early diagnosis of persistent asthma. Early childhood asthma diagnosis is relatively common. Unlike adult-onset asthma, many children diagnosed at a young age will have significant improvement in symptoms later as time passes, but others will not. Bose et al. developed machine learning models to identify which individuals diagnosed with asthma before age 5 continue to experience asthma-related visits [15]. Working with a retrospective EHR-based dataset for almost 10,000 children, they trained five machine learning models to differentiate patients without subsequent asthma-related visits (transient diagnosis) from those with asthma-related visits between ages 5 and 10 (persistent diagnosis). With good performance, they found that machine learning models could predict which individuals would experience persistent asthma. Efforts such as this may help guide clinician and parent decision-making in the early phases of pediatric asthma diagnosis.

These examples highlight some of the opportunities for future work aimed at early identification and intervention of childhood diseases, with the potential for AI to augment the practice of pediatric medicine.

Early risk prediction is another area in pediatric practice where the application of machine learning approaches can benefit patients, families, and their clinical providers in a full range of healthcare settings. Researchers, including pediatricians from the University of Utah, developed a model to predict hospital encounters for asthma in patients with a known asthma diagnosis [16]. Their final model reached a higher area under the curve on asthmatic adults vs. children, raising interesting questions about our understanding of the underlying disease process in children. Highlighting the fact that asthma in adults is different from asthma in children, it demonstrates the need for tailored approaches to risk prediction in pediatric populations. In another study, a novel, EHR-based predictive model was developed and validated as a population-level decision support tool for identifying children with complex health needs at high risk for future hospitalization [17]. In a different setting, one of the first large-scale studies to apply modern machine learning approaches specifically to a large emergency department (ED) population of children was able to improve discrimination ability during triage using only data that was routinely available at the time of triage, such as visit reason and vital signs [18]. In addition to predicting critical care and hospitalization, the models also achieved higher sensitivity for predicting the critical care outcome (meaning fewer under-triaged critically ill children) and higher specificity for predicting hospitalization outcome (fewer over triaged children who don't require inpatient care). This unique approach to better understanding how the commonly available variables the Emergency Department (ED) could be used to triage children in a more efficient and effective way sets a new standard for health informatics.

In the ED, particularly those that see fewer pediatric patients, time can be of the essence when making critical decisions. Trauma-related ED visits are relatively common, and efficient, timely assessment and management can be lifesaving. Niti Shahi et al. found that deep learning-based models, using a combination of clinical, laboratory, and radiographic features, can accurately predict the need for emergent intervention (massive transfusion or need for operative management) and mortality risk using data available in the first 4 hours [19]. While further research is needed to validate and understand the feasibility of applying this type of framework to a clinical setting, it underscores the value of early prediction, particularly for children who may require substantial periods of time to access subspecialty surgical intervention.

Likewise, a potential intervention-sparing application of machine learning models for clinical predictions and decision-making, a recent study demonstrated how machine learning-based predictive models using EHR data could predict children who are at low risk of spontaneous bacterial infection (SBI) and therefore may be spared unnecessary antibiotics and their associated adverse effects [20].

These use cases offer an encouraging view of how pediatric-specific initiatives further refinement of pediatric datasets could guide predictions and prompt decision support integration that promotes efficient and effective clinical management of young patients in the future.

Personalized Medicine

The application of AI in precision medicine for pediatric oncology is another of many areas in pediatric medicine that hold significant promise. While still in its early stages of discovery, considerable progress has been made to advance clinician tools in this space. For example, a recent study of late childhood cancer survivors demonstrated the potential value of a prediction model for anthracycline cardiotoxicity using a combination of genetic and clinical factors. Investigators determined that childhood cancer survivors with rare variants in specific genes have a lower susceptibility to anthracycline cardiotoxicity [21]. This demonstrates the potential value of a precision approach, with the hope that in the future, this technology can empower clinicians to optimize chemotherapy doses to maximize efficacy while minimizing the negative long-term effects of treatment.

Similarly, microRNA's (miRNA's), which help regulate cellular physiology, have been shown to play a role in various pediatric biological processes, from cancer and inflammation to neurodevelopmental disorders [22–24]. Chengyin et al. eloquently summarize some of the emerging research pairing patient miRNA-omics with longitudinal patient health data [25]. Understandably, in analyses of this kind, where data sets are large and complex, machine learning techniques can aid in the detection of biologically meaningful biomarkers that may potentially be therapeutic targets for pediatric diseases and precision care.

For various reasons to be discussed elsewhere in this chapter, pediatric AI research in precision medicine continues to lag behind that of adult patient populations. In order to achieve parity with adult AI applications, there must be awareness and advocacy for continued effort and investment in pediatric uses. Even in its infancy, precision medicine in pediatrics promises to improve pediatric health outcomes by providing a more specific and targeted approach to diagnosis and treatment based on each child's unique genetic, environmental, and lifestyle factors.

AI in Drug Development and Pharmacology

The use of AI in drug development and clinical pharmacology, more broadly, is an active area of investment and research. This effort can be particularly meaningful and simultaneously uniquely challenging for infants and children.

Compared with adults, most pediatric diseases affect small populations of children and thus are considered rare. This can lead to a lack of sufficient studies of drugs in these subgroups. Combining this with the relatively commonplace discontinuation and nonpublication of pediatric randomized controlled trials, it makes progress in the area of drug development for pediatric illness lag behind that of adults where blockbuster drugs are more likely to be brought to market [26]. A recent study by Yackey et al. observed that at least 1 drug was prescribed off-label in 28.1% of pediatric visits during their study period, with younger age, longer hospital stays, and mortality associated with higher rates of off-label use [27].

In this new era of increasingly large volumes of both structured and unstructured data captured longitudinally throughout infancy and childhood for younger patients, machine learning may have several useful potential applications in helping shape and direct the pharmacologic advancements in the pediatric population. Advanced predictive analytics can model diseases and associated treatments for infants and children in ways that haven't been seen before. Researchers at the University of Galway and Heidelberg University in Germany created 'digital babies' that can simulate infant metabolism in the first 6 months of life and predict known biomarkers for inherited metabolic diseases along with metabolic responses to various treatment strategies [28]. The authors suggest this could be a first step to digital metabolic twins for newborn infant metabolism, enabling tailored disease management for each infant's metabolic needs.

For pediatric clinical trials, AI could pool data from lower-volume disparate populations in efficient and effective ways. Likewise, the expansion of datasets to include less traditional data points, such as text from EHR notes, patient-reported data sourced from patient-facing apps, digital biomarkers, and even carefully crafted synthetic data could improve both the quantity and quality of clinical research initiatives. Nugent et al. describe a novel computational method that uses side-effect data mined from social media to inform computational drug repositioning to also potentially address the problem of side-effect under-reporting [29].

Understanding the multidimensional interactions of all types of blended data and how to safely and ethically leverage it on behalf of designing new pediatric pharmaceutical opportunities requires sharp attention to the risks as well. In the future, we can expect that high-quality data can take on many forms. Still, its utility is dependent on the prioritization of thoughtful data governance frameworks to address inconsistencies and inaccurate information, the establishment of transparent algorithms for building trust, dissipation of segregated data silos to generate larger volume data sets and streamlining and interoperability of fragmented electronic health data systems. We must simultaneously maintain patient privacy, translate effectively across disciplines, and safeguard against further contributing to bias, as the consequences for infants and children can be both severe and lifelong.

Enhancing Clinical Decision Support Systems (CDSS)

Clinical decision support systems (CDSS) are one area of focus for improving pediatric patient management and care. Many EHR systems already seamlessly integrate CDSS into its electronic health record, offering features like rules-based drug interaction alerts, best practice advisories, and chronic disease management protocols. The performance of these systems may be further enhanced by the utilization of machine learning-based algorithms to improve their predictive accuracy. And because pediatric diseases are not typically represented in large portions of the population, using AI to provide real-time decision support based on larger consolidated data sets has the potential to support clinicians in their effort to maximize diagnostic accuracy and treatment outcomes.

That said, there are essential challenges specific to pediatric-focused tools for pediatric applications of CDSS, including the limited sharing of data sets that accurately represent disease and patient diversity for effective modeling, a wide range of developmental variation across the pediatric patient continuum, along with important ethical, equity and medicolegal risks among other challenges [30]. With careful design and implementation, it is possible for traditional CDSS to evolve into useful and effective AI-driven tools.

Consider the specific potential value of AI-powered image analysis. Skin rashes are a staple in pediatric practice, starting with the earliest days of parental worry in the first newborn weeks through the dermatologic challenges of puberty. Drs. Castelo-Soccio and McMahon suggest that up to 30% of pediatric primary care visits involve skin-related problems, and one five-year multicenter review found that 3.3% of all emergency department visits were for general skin complaints, with only 4% of these requiring admission [31, 32]. Some rashes are true emergencies that require prompt diagnosis and treatment. With a shortage of pediatric dermatologists for both adequate training and consultation, AI stands to augment primary and urgent care in a truly meaningful way. Used in collaboration with clinical expertise, visual diagnostic tools have the potential to assist clinicians in making more efficient decisions about the diagnosis and treatment of various skin conditions.

Patient-Facing Tools and Applications

Active research and development suggest that future areas of scientific focus and potential commercial investment will include the use of AI in patient-facing, smartphone-based tools and applications for young patients and their families. Such technologies, while still never be a replacement for the human experience in healthcare, do have the potential to increase health engagement, early screening, and better access to information and services that can improve well-being and health literacy, while enhancing health data and health behavior visibility that can clear the way for earlier, more convenient diagnosis and management (reference). Neonatal jaundice detection, symptom-checkers, at-home spirometry for chronic pulmonary disease management, early identification of autism, mental health screening, and non-invasive organ transplant home monitoring platforms are just a few examples of tools that are in the early stages of development and validation within pediatric patients [33–40]. As with other areas of pediatric health AI research, progress in this area is limited by small pediatric patient data sets, lack of financial investment and lack of awareness of the potential opportunity for this population, as well as ethical and regulatory challenges.

Virtual Health Assistants and Chatbots

Virtual health assistants and chatbots are another set of future AI supported tools to consider for caregivers and young patients, particularly at a time of predicted shortages in the pediatric workforce, with increasing demands on fewer numbers of clinicians available to support patient and caregiver needs. These types of tools can reduce burden by supporting basic patient engagement. Moreover, AI-powered assistants and chatbots have the potential to provide continuous support, with the ability to provide families with the evidence-based information they need to make more informed, timely health-related decisions while empowering them to improve their child's health and more efficiently access and navigate the healthcare system.

Phone calls from worried new parents are the norm in pediatric healthcare. However, many parents struggle to access the information they need within our current structure of healthcare delivery, particularly those in areas of provider shortages, and have difficulty accessing timely connection to the information they need. Reports have detailed ED overuse in the setting of neonatal conditions, with the opportunity to close the gap through immediately responsive, same-day help and advice [41]. In one pilot study, a question-and-answer chatbot for new mothers of color demonstrated acceptable, feasible, and appropriate advice and intervention for ethnic and racial minority pregnant women and mothers of infants [42]. Its success lies in its ability to provide a personalized, flexible experience that increases the timeliness and accessibility of high-quality health information. While this type of innovation is in its infancy, and clinical trials ongoing, this use of AI holds great promise for the future support and fact-based guidance of new parents.

Wearable Devices and Remote Monitoring

Another aspect of how AI can influence pediatric care and management is through the use of medical devices and wearables. The pediatric devices on the market can be used to improve patient care outside of the hospital setting. For example, wearable technologies allow patients' vital signs to be monitored at home with data shared directly with healthcare providers. FDA-approved devices include AION's iTempShield for monitoring temperature in patients over five years old, and Gabi SmartCare's digital health platform provides real-time monitoring of children 0–12 years old through the wearing of a connected bracelet [43, 44]. Several technologies are using AI to improve how care is provided for children with asthma, including 'smart' stethoscopes like StethoMe that use AI to detect wheezing, [45] Other technologies can monitor pediatric seizures by wearing a watch and notifying caregivers [46].

Telemedicine and Telehealth

Finally, a discussion of the value of AI in the management and care of pediatric patients would not be complete without the review of patient-facing AI-enhanced telemedicine platforms. The COVID-19 pandemic inspired a rapid expansion of telehealth services by pediatricians and subspecialists, permanently impacting many aspects of healthcare delivery models worldwide [47]. The pandemic inspired the rapid development of telehealth systems within pediatric patient portals, allowing for continued study of both the value, such as increasing access to care, and potential risks of virtual care technology, like privacy, cost, and challenges related to health equity and the digital divide [48, 49]. Considering these risks when applying machine learning technology to telehealth systems is essential. Machine learning models can be burdened by similar challenges, potentially magnifying the already burdensome disparities within both local and global healthcare systems.

Still in the early stages, with limited examples in pediatrics, there is potential for successful pairing of AI with telehealth. Foster et al. describe examples of remote patient monitoring. A form of telemedicine, remote patient monitoring can promote proactive clinical management and patient and caregiver engagement, particularly for pediatric chronic disease management [50]. Citing examples for cardiac rhythm, Type 1 diabetes, and asthma control, they underscored the need for integrated models of pediatric care that include valuable data collected outside of the traditional office environment. As an example, TytoCare has created a pediatric telehealth platform that allows families to use a stethoscope, otoscope, and camera to evaluate the heart and lungs, ears and throat, and skin, respectively [51]. Currently, Boston Children's Hospital is using TytoCare in select clinics [52]. If integrated carefully, AI-enhanced telemedicine using tools such as risk prediction, remote monitoring, symptom triage, and decision support systems have the potential to refine our approach to alternate models of patient-focused care delivery.

Future Directions

There is immense promise for AI to advance patient care in pediatrics. It is imperative for companies to continue to innovate and invest in pediatric technologies. AI for pediatric medical applications requires research and development that considers patients' biological, developmental, and psychosocial needs from birth through adulthood. Pediatric experts must be embedded in the cross-disciplinary efforts of health AI innovation to safely and productively navigate the nuanced impact of what is being designed and built on behalf of advancing pediatric clinical outcomes and population health.

References

1. Fischer GA, Wells SM, Rebuffoni JF, Peterson BM, LeBien TW. A model for overcoming challenges in academic pediatric medical device innovation. J Clin Transl Sci. 2019;3(1):5–11.
2. Nundy S, Cooper LA, Mate KS. The quintuple aim for health care improvement: a new imperative to advance health equity. Institute for Healthcare Improvement. https://www.ihi.org/resources/publications/quintuple-aim-health-care-improvement-new-imperative-advance-health-equity. Accessed 5 June 2024.
3. Hackett M. The pediatrics field lags in digital innovations, but a new accelerator is looking to change that paradigm. MobiHealthNews. September 3, 2020. https://www.mobihealthnews.com/news/pediatrics-field-lags-digital-innovations-new-accelerator-looking-change-paradigm. Accessed 5 June 2024.
4. Dey T, Gaskin C, Khurana B, et al. The role of artificial intelligence in pediatric radiology: current status and future prospects. J Am Coll Radiol. 2023;20(8):1178–85.
5. Davendralingam N, Sebire NJ, Arthurs OJ, Shelmerdine SC. Artificial intelligence in paediatric radiology: future opportunities. Br J Radiol. 2021;94(1117):20200975.
6. Radiating hope: expanding AI in pediatric radiology for a brighter future. American College of Radiology. July 28, 2023. Available at: https://www.acr.org/Advocacy-and-Economics/Voice-of-Radiology-Blog/2023/07/28/Expanding-AI-in-Pediatric-Radiology-for-a-Brighter-Future. Accessed 11 June 2024.
7. Contrive Datum Insights. AI in medical imaging market is projected to reach US$ 20.9 billion by 2030 at a CAGR of 36.87% during the forecast period 2023–2030. GlobeNewswire. https://www.globenewswire.com/news-release/2023/01/25/2594827/0/en/AI-in-Medical-Imaging-Market-is-projected-to-Reach-US-20-9-Billion-by-2030-at-a-CAGR-of-36-87-during-the-forecast-period-2023-2030-Contrive-Datum-Insights.html. Published January 25, 2023. Accessed 19 June 2024.
8. Clark MM, Hildreth A, Batalov S, Ding Y, Chowdhury S, Watkins K, et al. Diagnosis of genetic diseases in seriously ill children by rapid whole-genome sequencing and automated phenotyping and interpretation. Sci Transl Med. 2019;11(489):eaat6177.
9. Meng F, Li F, Wu S, Yang T, Xiao Z, Zhang Y, et al. Machine learning-based early diagnosis of autism according to eye movements of real and artificial faces scanning. Front Neurosci. 2023;17:1170951. Published 2023 Sep 15.
10. Jeyarani A, Senthikumar R. Eye tracking biomarkers for autism spectrum disorder detection using machine learning and deep learning techniques: review. Res Autism Spectr Disord. 2023;108(4):102228.
11. Abbas H, Garberson F, Liu-Mayo S, Glover E, Wall DP. Multi-modular AI approach to streamline autism diagnosis in young children. Sci Rep. 2020;10(5014). https://doi.org/10.1038/s41598-020-61213-w.
12. Cheng ER, Steinhardt R, Ben Miled Z. Predicting childhood obesity using machine learning: practical considerations. BioMedInformatics. 2022;2(1):184–203.
13. Qin H, Zhang L, Li X, Xu Z, Zhang J, Wang S, Zheng L, et al. Pediatric obstructive sleep apnea diagnosis: leveraging machine learning with linear discriminant analysis. Front Neurosci. 2024;12:1328209. Published 2024 Feb 14.
14. Lure AC, Du X, Black EW, Irons R, Lemas DJ, Taylor JA, et al. Using machine learning analysis to assist in differentiating between necrotizing enterocolitis and spontaneous intestinal perforation: a novel predictive analytic tool. J Pediatr Surg. 2021;56(10):1703–10. https://doi.org/10.1016/j.jpedsurg.2020.11.008.
15. Bose S, Kenyon CC, Masino AJ. Personalized prediction of early childhood asthma persistence: a machine learning approach. PLoS One. 2021;16(3):e0247784.
16. Luo G, He S, Stone BL, Nkoy FL, Johnson MD. Developing a model to predict hospital encounters for asthma in asthmatic patients: secondary analysis. JMIR Med Inform. 2020;8(1):e16080.

17. Ming DY, Zhao C, Tang X, Chung RJ, Rogers UA, Stirling A, et al. Predictive modeling to identify children with complex health needs at risk for hospitalization. Hosp Pediatr. 2023;13(5):357–69.
18. Goto T, Camargo CA, Faridi MK, Freishtat RJ, Hasegawa K. Machine learning–based prediction of clinical outcomes for children during emergency department triage. JAMA Netw Open. 2019;2(1):e186937.
19. Shahi N, Shahi A. Decision-making in pediatric blunt solid organ injury: a deep learning approach to predict massive transfusion, need for operative management, and mortality risk. J Pediatr Surg. 2020;56(2):379–84.
20. Martin B, DeWitt P, Scott HF, Parker S, Bennett TD. Machine learning approach to predicting absence of serious bacterial infection at PICU admission. Hosp Pediatr. 2022;12(6):590–603.
21. Chaix M, Parmar N, Kinnear C, Lafreniere-Roula M, Akinrinade O, Yao R, et al. Machine learning identifies clinical and genetic factors associated with anthracycline cardiotoxicity in pediatric cancer survivors. J Am Coll Cardiol CardioOnc. 2020;2(5):690–706.
22. Peng Y, Croce C. The role of MicroRNAs in human cancer. Sig Transduct Target Ther. 2016;1:15004.
23. Batra SK, Heier CR, Diaz-Calderon L, Tully CB, Fiorillo AA, van den Anker J, et al. Serum miRNAs are pharmacodynamic biomarkers associated with therapeutic response in pediatric inflammatory bowel disease. Inflamm Bowel Dis. 2020;26(10):1597–606.
24. Hicks SD, Ignacio C, Gentile K, Middleton FA. Salivary miRNA profiles identify children with autism spectrum disorder, correlate with adaptive behavior, and implicate ASD candidate genes involved in neurodevelopment. BMC Pediatr. 2016;16:52. Published 2016 Apr 22
25. Li C, Sullivan RE, Zhu D, Hicks SD. Putting the "mi" in omics: discovering miRNA biomarkers for pediatric precision care. Pediatr Res. 2022;93:316–23. https://doi.org/10.1038/s41390-022-02206-5.
26. Pica N, Bourgeois F. Discontinuation and nonpublication of randomized clinical trials conducted in children. Pediatrics. 2016;138(3):e20160223.
27. Yackey K, Stukus K, Cohen D, Kline D, Zhao S, Stanley R. Off-label medication prescribing patterns in pediatrics: an update. Hosp Pediatr. 2019;9(3):186–93.
28. Zaunseder E, Mütze U, Okun JG, Hoffmann GF, Kölker S, Heuveline V, et al. Personalized metabolic whole-body models for newborns and infants predict growth and biomarkers of inherited metabolic diseases. Cell Metab. 2024;36:1–16.
29. Plachouras V, Leidner JL, et al. Quantifying self-reported adverse drug events on Twitter: signal and topic analysis. In: Proceedings of the 7th 2016 International conference on social media & society; 6 Feb 2016.
30. Youssef A, Ng MY, Long J, Hernandez-Boussard T, Shah N, Miner A, et al. Organizational factors in clinical data sharing for artificial intelligence in health care. JAMA Netw Open. 2023;6(12):e2348422.
31. Castelo-Soccio L, McMahon P. Pediatric dermatology. J Clin Aesthet Dermatol. 2017;10(3):S8–S15.
32. Baibergenova A, Shear NH. Skin conditions that bring patients to emergency departments. Arch Dermatol. 2011;147(1):118–20. https://doi.org/10.1001/archdermatol.2010.246.
33. Jiménez-Díaz G, Aune A, Elizarrarás-Rivas J, Gierman LM, Keitsch M, Marcuzzi A, et al. Neonatal jaundice detection in low-resource Mexican settings: possibilities and barriers for innovation with mobile health. BMC Health Serv Res. 2024;24(1):671.
34. Jazayeri SMH, Jamshidnezhad A. Top mobile applications in pediatrics and children's health: assessment and intelligent analysis tools for a systematic investigation. Malays J Med Sci. 2019;26(1):5–14.
35. Benoit JRA, Hartling L, Scott SD. Bridging evidence-to-care gaps with mHealth: Designing a symptom checker for parents accessing knowledge translation resources on acute children's illnesses in a smartphone application. PEC Innov. 2023;2:100152.

36. Kruizinga MD, Essers E, Stuurman FE, Zhuparris A, van Eik N, Janssens HM, et al. Technical validity and usability of a novel smartphone-connected spirometry device for pediatric patients with asthma and cystic fibrosis. Pediatr Pulmonol. 2020;55(9):2463–70.
37. Van Sickle D, Barrett M, Humblet O, Henderson K, Hogg C. Randomized, controlled study of the impact of a mobile health tool on asthma SABA use, control, and adherence. Eur Respir J. 2016;48:PA1018.
38. Chang Z, Di Martino JM, Aiello R, Baker J, Carpenter K, Compton S, et al. Computational methods to measure patterns of gaze in toddlers with autism spectrum disorder. JAMA Pediatr. 2021;175(8):827–36.
39. O'Leary A, Lahey T, Loftness B, Douglas A, Skelton J, et al. Using wearable digital devices to screen children for mental health conditions: ethical promises and challenges. Sensors (Basel). 2024;24(10):3214.
40. Adib R, Das D, Ahamed SI, Lerret SM. An mHealth app-based self-management intervention for family members of pediatric transplant recipients (myFAMI): framework design and development study. JMIR Nurs. 2022;5(1):e32785.
41. Harrold J, Langevin M, for the Pediatric Emergency Research Canada Network, et al. Parental characteristics and perspectives pertaining to neonatal visits to the emergency department: a multicentre survey. CMAJ Open. 2018;6(3):E423–9.
42. Nguyen QC, Aparicio EM, Jasczynski M, Channell Doig A, Yue X, Mane H, et al. Rosie, a health education question-and-answer chatbot for new mothers: randomized pilot study. JMIR Form Res. 2024;8. https://doi.org/10.2196/51361.
43. FDA approves AION's iTempShield Device and Software System. Medical Device Network. August 31, 2023. https://www.medicaldevice-network.com/news/fda-aion-itempshield-device-software/. Accessed 23 June 2024.
44. Gabi SmartCare obtains FDA certification to market its digital pediatric solutions in the United States. Business Wire. January 8, 2024. https://www.businesswire.com/news/home/20240108595274/en/Gabi-SmartCare-Obtains-FDA-Certification-to-Market-Its-Digital-Pediatric-Solutions-in-the-United-States. Accessed 23 June 2024.
45. Newman T. New at-home stethoscope may improve home monitoring of asthma in young children. Medical News Today. February 26, 2024. https://www.medicalnewstoday.com/articles/new-at-home-stethoscope-may-improve-home-monitoring-of-asthma-in-young-children. Accessed 23 June 2024.
46. Cerretani J. Predicting pediatric seizures with a wristband: Study shows what's possible. Boston Children's Answers. February 2, 2021. https://answers.childrenshospital.org/seizure-tracking/. Accessed 23 June 2024.
47. Katzow MW, Steinway C, Jan S. Telemedicine and health disparities during COVID-19. Pediatrics. 2020;146(2):e20201586.
48. Patel PD, Cobb J, Wright D, Turer RW, Jordan T, Humphrey A, et al. Rapid development of telehealth capabilities within pediatric patient portal infrastructure for COVID-19 care: barriers, solutions, results. J Am Med Inform Assoc. 2020;27(7):1116–20.
49. Kuziemsky C, Hunter I, Udayasankaran JG, Ranatunga P, Kulatunga G, John S, et al. Telehealth as a means of enabling health equity. Yearb Med Inform. 2022;31(1):60–6.
50. Foster C, Schinasi D, Kan K, Macy M, Wheeler D, Curfman A. Remote monitoring of patient- and family-generated health data in pediatrics. Pediatrics. 2022;149(2):e2021054137. https://doi.org/10.1542/peds.2021-054137.
51. The best pediatric telehealth platforms for kids—and moms. TytoCare. November 10, 2021. https://www.tytocare.com/consumers/news-and-events/the-best-pediatric-telehealth-platforms-for-kids-and-moms/. Accessed 23 June 2024.
52. Digital Health, TytoCare. Boston Children's Hospital. https://www.childrenshospital.org/digital-health/tytocare. Accessed 23 June 2024.

Chapter 8
Artificial Intelligence in Pediatric Healthcare: Unique Considerations

Amy Molten and Alyssa Abo

Unique Considerations for AI in Pediatrics

Pediatric Population Health

Pediatric-specific population health represents unique challenges and opportunities distinct from adult-focused approaches, primarily due to the dynamic nature of infant, child and adolescent monitoring and intervention. The rapidly changing processes that inform physical, developmental, and behavioral health and wellbeing in the pediatric population requires that healthcare strategies and AI models continually adapt to age- and development-specific norms and milestones that are not linear nor uniformly predictable. This can potentially exacerbate the already complex machine learning challenges of the smaller or imbalanced datasets in younger age groups, affecting reliability and generalizability of models, and limiting the development and implementation of pediatric population health initiatives.

Nevertheless, if done carefully, the application of AI in pediatric population health holds significant potential for advancing initiatives in pediatric care. For example, the detection and management of rare diseases take on added significance in pediatrics. Although by definition a rare disease affects a small number of individuals, at the population level there are estimated to be more than 7000 identified types in existence, affecting approximately 300 million people worldwide [2]. Given that almost 70% of rare disease presents in childhood, rapid, early diagnosis can enhance lifetime health outcomes and quality of life, while reducing both treatment costs and the incidence of financial hardship related to rare diseases [2, 3].

A. Molten
Department of Pediatrics, Tufts Medical Center, Boston, MA, USA

A. Abo (✉)
Impact1 at Stanford Mussallem Center for Biodesign, Stanford Medicine, Stanford, CA, USA

T. Adirim (ed.), *Digital Health, AI and Generative AI in Healthcare*,
https://doi.org/10.1007/978-3-031-83526-1_8

Likewise, emphasizing opportunity in behavioral and mental health, AI-assisted assessment tools and interventions, with a particular focus on early detection of neurodevelopmental disorders, can have lifelong impacts on entire populations of children and adolescents [4]. And the integration of pediatric health data with educational and social services in could address the holistic needs of children. AI technologies could play a vital role in early detection and management of various physical, developmental, and behavioral health issues through the application of school-based health screening and intervention programs that closely align with primary care systems.

Vaccination and immunization strategies take on heightened importance in pediatric population health, with AI tools potentially optimizing schedules, predicting outbreak risks, and combating disinformation to ensure timely and comprehensive coverage. UNICEF and other global organizations are actively working to harness AI for global health equity through vaccine-focused projects, working to leverage artificial intelligence and digital health to support public health initiatives for children [5].

Pediatric-focused AI systems of this kind must be developed and deployed responsibly, with robust frameworks and safeguards to maintain public trust in these technologies and pediatric medicine more broadly. For the youngest patients, mistrust could fuel AI skepticism, as seen with immunization campaigns, limiting positive progress for future generations [6]. Such significant social impact risks require AI developers, clinicians, policymakers, ethicists, and patients and families to carefully and thoughtfully proactively address these implications to ensure pediatric AI benefits children and society equitably. Close interdisciplinary collaboration, responsible research and analytics frameworks, and attention to the unique developmental, behavioral, educational, family, environmental, and ethical considerations of pediatric patients, prioritization of pediatric population health initiatives can provide valuable insights that promote the well-being of infants, children, and adolescents at the population level.

Health Literacy

One area of important consideration is the use of AI tools to increase pediatric patient and family health literacy. *Healthy People 2030* defines health literacy as the degree to which individuals can to find, understand, and use information and services to inform health-related decisions and actions for themselves and others [7]. The most recent population-level estimates from a National Assessment of Adult Literacy survey suggest that only 12% of Americans have proficient health literacy, disproportionately impacting populations of color [8]. And over one-third of US adults would have difficulty with common health tasks, such as following directions on a prescription drug label or adhering to a childhood immunization schedule using a standard chart [8]. In pediatrics, this raises concerns about the caregiver's ability to guide children in daily health-decision making or understand a child's symptoms to make effective health decisions when their child is sick.

Effective use of AI to improve health literacy for adults and children is still in the early stages of development. Interactive conversational systems like Siri or ChatGPT are readily available to consumers to answer questions and increase their understanding of health topics. However, biases and potential amplification of misinformation prevent their effective use for addressing large-scale health literacy challenges. Nonetheless, AI has potential to enhance health literacy, and potentially longer-term value if aiming these tools and interventions for children and adolescents [9, 10]. One randomized controlled trial, a mobile video game embedded with implicit learning components showed a strong positive impact on children's food choices immediately following the game [11]. While still in the early phases of development, and although additional and longer-term studies are needed to understand the impact on overall health literacy, educational AI games, intelligent tutoring systems, personalized conversational agents, customized health communications, and other applications do hold significant potential for AI-powered technology to engage children and their families in building health knowledge over time.

Health Equity, Access, and Engagement

Early research suggests that AI can play a role in identifying and understanding patterns of child health risks and disparities, as well as potentially addressing inequalities by improving access to health services [12–14]. Likewise, there is an opportunity to use AI to help mitigate care barriers for higher-risk populations, and potentially close education, language and access gaps to promote health equity [15, 16]. Consider adolescent patients, who are particularly susceptible to engaging in behaviors that could put their health and well-being at risk. It is well known that they may also be reluctant to consult their healthcare providers, especially about sensitive or potentially stigmatizing issues. And in the age of electronic medical record recording, a layer of additional concern about unintentional disclosures to caregivers is added to this already strained communication. A team from Stanford Medicine Children's Health is investigating how a large language model could help prevent disclosures of sensitive information by identifying confidential content within adolescents' clinical notes [17]. As generative AI becomes more ubiquitous in healthcare; the range of potential utility continues to expand. These solutions intended to promote health equity and access must be developed with great care for data integrity and responsible, inclusive design to avoid bias and worsening of disparities.

Evidence also suggests that AI holds promise for predicting outcomes of behavior change interventions and resource access and utilization, potentially paving the way for an entirely new way of engaging with patients in positive health behavior change, even in areas of provider or health resource shortages [18, 19]. This, combined with relatively universal mobile phone usage worldwide, is unlocking entirely new areas of research for children and their caregivers.

Pediatric Healthcare Operations

While most of the operational and administrative innovation is designed to be generalizable to the full range of provider, health system and hospital types, there is certainly opportunity to consider tools that are specifically aligned with pediatric patients and their caregivers needs.

For example, body weight is a critical pediatric vital sign for infants and children, requiring accurate documentation by clinical staff not just as a visual representation of growth and development patterns, but also as an important safety metric for medication dose calculation. Medication dosing errors are more common in pediatrics because of weight-based dosing calculation requirements [20]. Researchers at Cincinnati Children's Hospital Medical Center developed a machine learning-based automated weight abnormality detector to analyze growth dynamics in pediatric weight charts and detect abnormal weight values, with the potential to support safer care delivery that relies on accurate and reliable weight measures [21].

A team at Boston Children's Hospital developed a deep learning-based approach for predicting the risk of no-shows when a medical appointment is first scheduled. While their intuitive results found past no-show records as the strongest predictor of future behavior, a better understanding of unique patterns of a pediatric patient population can serve as a guide for anticipating and intervening in targeted ways [22].

Ambient AI listening technology is an active area of research and development, taking notes and generating a written summary that captures the essential clinical details for healthcare providers to boost the provider-patient relationship and decrease administrative burden. In pediatric medicine, there are unique considerations for successful implementation. To start, the technology would need to be able to detect and accurately interpret vocalizations, speech patterns and language skills for the full range of ages and developmental stages. While we can imagine a world where the technology itself may be able to support the early identification of developmental delay or pediatric disorders, such as speech and language delays, autism spectrum disorder or hearing impairment, this capability remains far into the future.

Ambient AI listening naturally raises significant privacy concerns, and while strict protocols should be in place to protect patient and family privacy, the technology itself may create a barrier to effective interviews, particularly with adolescent patients. Interviewing in medicine can be fragile, with trust-building at the center of a relationship between the adolescent patient and the adult provider. With sensitive details being recorded throughout, it will be essential to understand how this technology may impact patient disclosure of important details of their immediate medical and emotional health needs or affect their willingness to seek care. This holds true with the utilization of large language models to help clinicians draft messages to patients, which can be an efficient form of communication with adolescent minors who have health record and provider communication autonomy but would be an especially vulnerable group in the setting of unintended data disclosures.

These are just a handful of specific considerations for the responsible and effective implementation of intelligent automation in pediatric healthcare settings. We must ensure that our innovation efforts enhance provider systems and optimize patient care while prioritizing safety, ethics, and developmental appropriateness.

Pediatric- Specific Ethical, Legal, and Social Implications

The use of AI in pediatric populations raises vital and specific ethical, legal, and social implications that must be carefully considered when designing and implementing new approaches to pediatric care delivery.

The US Surgeon General's 2024 call for a warning label on social media platforms represents an important example of the critical ethical responsibilities faced in technology [23]. The untoward public health risks are not to be taken lightly and require heightened attention as efforts are made to integrate technology and machine learning into healthcare [24–27]. As we work to develop new and better approaches to improving healthcare delivery and experience, it is important to balance the unique ethical considerations for pediatric patients with the financial incentives generated by the multibillion-dollar venture capital investments in healthcare AI.

As discussed in Chap. 10, the principle of beneficence, one of the core ethical principles in healthcare, refers to the obligation to act in the patient's best interest and minimize harm. This is especially true for children, who are vulnerable members of society due to their range of cognitive and decisional abilities and dependence on adults for care, decision-making, and consent. This heightens the obligation of health and technology professionals to act in their best interest and prioritize their well-being. Likewise, the definition of 'best interest' of an infant, child, or adolescent can be more complex than that of adults who can express their individual health preferences. Focus for young patients must extend beyond their medical factors to include the developmental, emotional, psychosocial, and family variables that can affect both risks and benefits associated with innovation. Social media is an example of technological innovation whose design challenges the principle of beneficence. It highlights the need for a heightened level of responsibility when innovating on behalf of pediatric patients, with robust human clinician oversight and scientific judgment to ensure AI systems are aligned with humanistic values to preserve well-being.

Privacy and data security rights are other important ethical considerations in the development of AI applications as discussed in Chap. 12. AI solutions developed for adults using adult data are not necessarily generalizable across the entire age spectrum because of pediatric patients' physiologic, anatomical, and developmental differences. However, children account for a smaller proportion of healthcare resources and associated clinical and research data, leading to smaller AI model training datasets that may not be sufficiently robust or free of bias. Smaller datasets can also raise significant privacy concerns, requiring more resilient de-identification techniques and data governance frameworks to protect sensitive attributes of this vulnerable population.

The potential consequences of privacy violations can be severe and lifelong. Compromised confidentiality of sensitive medical and personal information for a minor could lead to possible discrimination or stigmatization in the future based on their health conditions or disabilities. Insufficient protection of children's privacy and data when adopting new health technologies could negatively and permanently impact their future social health, education, and employment potential.

Finally, as with data privacy and security, the lack of robust data to represent pediatric populations can lead to bias and underrepresentation in the AI algorithms for young patients, particularly those across dimensions such as race, gender, socio-economic status, and disabilities. For example, without adequate representation in a dataset, a patient query of limb pain and cough through an AI-powered symptom-checking tool may fail to surface vaso-occlusion precipitating acute chest syndrome, a leading cause of hospitalization and death in people with sickle cell disease. Requiring early diagnosis and treatment, an error of this type could delay care and treatment and perpetuate or exacerbate existing health disparities.

Biases and unfair data practices in healthcare can have significant consequences for adult health outcomes, quality of life, and life expectancy. Still, the impacts are likely to be short-term compared to those experienced during critical developmental stages. In this pediatric population, lack of investment in fair and inclusive datasets and systems can have long-lasting negative impacts on their biopsychosocial development. Strategies for developing ethical AI in pediatric healthcare should include strong interdisciplinary collaboration and diverse perspectives in the earliest stages of development and ensuring fairness and inclusivity as crucial design principles from the outset. Furthermore, rigorous bias testing, strict data governance and auditing of algorithms to identify and manage potential sources of bias or unfairness should be a minimum standard when adopting new health technologies.

The design and deployment of AI systems in pediatric healthcare comes with significant legal and regulatory considerations. As described above, the vulnerability of pediatric populations, combined with the potential long-term impacts on their health and well-being, requires careful implementation of AI in clinical practice.

Not all health AI vertices are subject to current regulatory oversight, and there is an urgent need to develop child-centered artificial intelligence policies in healthcare and technology more broadly. While many academic and pharmaceutical projects are subject to specific governing body standards, such as the US Food and Drug Administration, healthcare AI regulations in the US vary in scope, with an expanding compilation of laws and rules visible at the local, state, and federal levels (see Chap. 14). The lack of consistent, centralized governance and monitoring allows risk of developers using swift but potentially reckless data practices at the expense of quality and patient safety. Inconsistent validation standards add to the challenges of scientifically grounded progress in healthcare AI.

Consider a study from early 2024, where researchers from Cohen Children's Medical Center examined the diagnostic accuracy of a large language model in pediatric case studies [28]. Not surprisingly, ChatGPT version 3.5 reached an incorrect diagnosis in 83% of pediatric case challenges. What remains concerning, however, is that this tool is free and publicly available to all, including to those without the clinical training required to understand when results are true or false. The overwhelmingly inaccurate diagnostic performance of this and other active patient-facing chatbots underscores the invaluable role that regulatory boundaries and governance processes hold. While potentially slowing the warp-speed pace of technological innovation in healthcare, they play a crucial part in promoting transparency, accountability, and trust in the use of AI for children's healthcare.

Clear guidelines and standards must be established for transparent reporting of the AI platform's methodology and explainability, data sources, and potential limitations of clinical use. In addition, mechanisms for quality control, including regularly updating and revalidating the system as new datas becomes available or as patients evolve over time, must also be implemented with appropriate regulatory oversight to ensure the safety and well-being of vulnerable pediatric patient populations.

Conclusion

Machine learning and generative AI offer excellent possibilities for augmenting pediatric care delivery, designing new ways to address the unique needs of infants, children, adolescents, and their caregivers, and improving child health outcomes. These chapters highlight some of the ways machine learning and AI is being explored and implemented across various areas within the pediatric medicine domain, as well as the distinct characteristics of pediatric populations that necessitate a careful, purposeful approach to child health innovations.

Some basic guiding principles have emerged from the remarkable efforts to bring new science and technology to this rapidly evolving field. These and future learnings can hopefully be carefully applied to future initiatives:

1. Guidance and care by specially trained humans are the cornerstone of a holistic approach to pediatric medicine. While our physiological, behavioral, and emotional well-being can be relatively patterned, we each have our unique barriers to achieving an ideal state of health. This is especially true for infants and children, who live a complex interplay of evolving physiology, distinct disease patterns, developmental susceptibilities, dependence on caregivers for emotional support and decision-making, and variable communication skills. This makes pediatric patients even more vulnerable and susceptible to machine learning missteps, especially when assumptions are made about turning algorithms and products trained on adult data toward the pediatric population. The design, training, validation, and implementation of AI in pediatrics requires distinct approaches from those used for adults, such that researchers and developers must proceed with care.
2. While data production in healthcare is complex and high volume, infants and children account for a smaller proportion of clinical and research data, leading to more limited training data availability. Smaller datasets increase the risk of poor

performance, bias, ethical concerns and privacy challenges. There are various strategies that researchers and developers in pediatric AI can use when working with low-volume data; ultimately, they should strive to ensure that the resulting applications are meticulously evaluated and validated to promote beneficence and minimize harm.

3. Ethical issues are important in pediatric medicine and are potentially more complex because of a child's dependence on adults for care, consent, and decision-making. For this reason, applications of AI in pediatric healthcare must be both patient- and family-centered for successful implementation, and strategy and development teams should include contributors with deep clinical practice experience to ensure accuracy, safety, and utility in the real world.
4. Despite the explosion of AI-enabled innovation in healthcare, there remains a profound need for more investment in pediatrics. Children account for almost a quarter of the US population, and despite this, pediatric healthcare has been chronically overlooked and underfunded by both private and public sectors. With a strong commitment to including children in these innovation efforts, we can avoid perpetuating and even worsening the already existing gaps in child health and health outcomes. This could have both short-term and lifelong societal consequences. We have an opportunity to rethink this approach and consider how prioritizing AI development and deployment in this population could ensure that all people can benefit equally from advancement in healthcare AI, and positively impact the care that young patients receive today and into the future.
5. The rapidly evolving landscape of AI in healthcare needs to have governance mechanisms for developing and using AI technologies in healthcare. And the distinct characteristics of pediatric populations require tailored approaches to developing regulation and policies to guide its use. The lack of a unified approach to safe, equitable, ethical, and effective development and implementation of these emerging technologies limits our opportunity for positively advancing the patient and family experience, pediatric population health outcomes, healthcare costs, and provider satisfaction. A deliberate, coordinated, interdisciplinary and collaborative approach to pediatric AI policy should leverage the tremendous subject matter expertise within the pediatric community, including patients and their families, to establish robust, trustful industry and legislative partnerships to swiftly address the unique ethical, legal, financial, and data considerations for innovation in pediatric medicine.

References

1. Nundy S, Cooper LA, Mate KS. The quintuple aim for health care improvement: a new imperative to advance health equity. Institute for Healthcare Improvement. https://www.ihi.org/resources/publications/quintuple-aim-health-care-improvement-new-imperative-advance-health-equity. Accessed 5 June 2024.
2. The Lancet Global Health. The landscape for rare diseases in 2024. Lancet Glob Health. 2024;12(3):e341.

3. Chung CCY, Ng NYT, Ng YNC, Lui ACY, Fung JLF, Chan MCY, et al. Socio-economic costs of rare diseases and the risk of financial hardship: a cross-sectional study. Lancet Reg Health West Pac. 2023;34:100711.
4. Barua PD, Vicnesh J, Gururajan R, Oh SL, Palmer E, Azizan MM, et al. Artificial intelligence enabled personalised assistive tools to enhance education of children with neurodevelopmental disorders-a review. Int J Environ Res Public Health. 2022;19(3):1192. Published 2022 Jan 21.
5. Kallander, K. Digital for zero-dose: Harnessing AI for Global Health Equity. UNICEF. https://www.unicef.org/blog/digital-zero-dose-harnessing-ai-global-health-equity. Published June 2024. Accessed Aug 2024.
6. Neely SR, Eldredge C, Ersing R, Remington C. Vaccine hesitancy and exposure to misinformation: a survey analysis. J Gen Intern Med. 2022;37(1):179–87.
7. US Department of Health and Human Services. Healthy People 2030. Office of Disease Prevention and Health Promotion. https://health.gov/healthypeople. Published 2020. Accessed June 2024.
8. Kutner M, Greenberg E, et al. The health literacy of America's adults: results from the 2003 National Assessment of Adult Literacy (NCES 2006-483). Washington, DC: U.S. Department of Education, National Center for Education Statistics; 2006.
9. Bickmore TW, Pfeifer LM, Byron D, Forsythe S, Henault LE, Jack BW, et al. Usability of conversational agents by patients with inadequate health literacy: evidence from two clinical trials. J Health Commun. 2010;15(Suppl 2):197–210.
10. Milne-Ives M, de Cock C, Lim E, Shehadeh MH, de Pennington N, Mole G, et al. The effectiveness of artificial intelligence conversational agents in health care: systematic review. J Med Internet Res. 2020;22(10):e20346.
11. Kato-Lin YC, Kumar UB, Sri Prakash B, Prakash B, Varadan V, Agnihotri S, et al. Impact of pediatric mobile game play on healthy eating behavior: randomized controlled trial. JMIR Mhealth Uhealth. 2020;8(11):e15717. Published 2020 Nov 18. https://doi.org/10.2196/15717.
12. Samuel O, Zewotir T, North D. Application of machine learning methods for predicting under-five mortality: analysis of Nigerian demographic health survey 2018 dataset. BMC Med Inform Decis Mak. 2024;24(1):86.
13. Xiao Y, Mann JJ, Chow JCC, Brown TT, Snowden LR, Yip PS, et al. Patterns of social determinants of health and child mental health, cognition, and physical health. JAMA Pediatr. 2023;177(12):1294–305.
14. Green BL, Murphy A, Robinson E. Accelerating health disparities research with artificial intelligence. Front Digit Health. 2024;6:1330160.
15. Smitherman LC, Golden WC, Walton JR. Health disparities and their effects on children and their caregivers during the coronavirus disease 2019 pandemic. Pediatr Clin N Am. 2021;68(5):1133–45.
16. Brewster RCL, Gonzalez P, Khazanchi R, Butler A, Selcer R, Chu D, et al. Performance of ChatGPT and Google Translate for pediatric discharge instruction translation. Pediatrics. 2024;154(1):e2023065573.
17. Sisk BA, Antes AL, DuBois JM. An overarching framework for the ethics of artificial intelligence in pediatrics. JAMA Pediatr. 2024;178(3):213–4.
18. Mac Aonghusa P, Michie S. Artificial intelligence and behavioral science through the looking glass: challenges for real-world application. Ann Behav Med. 2020;54(12):942–7.
19. Michie S, Thomas J, Mac Aonghusa P, West R, Johnston M, Kelly MP, et al. The Human Behaviour-Change Project: an artificial intelligence system to answer questions about changing behaviour. Wellcome Open Res. 2020;5:122.
20. The Joint Commission. Preventing pediatric medication errors—sentinel event alert. Complimentary Publication of the Joint Commission; April 2021. p. 39.
21. Liu L, Wu DTY, Spooner SA, Ni Y. Development and evaluation of an automated approach to detect weight abnormalities in pediatric weight charts. AMIA Annu Symp Proc. 2021;2021:783–92.

22. Liu D, Shin WY, Sprecher E, Conroy K, Santiago O, Wachtel G, et al. Machine learning approaches to predicting no-shows in pediatric medical appointment. NPJ Digit Med. 2022;5(1):50. Published 2022 Apr 20
23. US Surgeon General. Advisory on social media and youth mental health. US Department of Health and Human Services; 2023.
24. Riehm KE, Feder KA, Tormohlen KN, Crum RM, Young AS, Green KM, et al. Associations between time spent using social media and internalizing and externalizing problems among US youth. JAMA Psychiatry. 2019;76(12):1266–73.
25. Memon AM, Sharma SG, Mohite SS, Jain S. The role of online social networking on deliberate self-harm and suicidality in adolescents: a systematized review of literature. Indian J Psychiatry. 2018;60(4):384–92.
26. Kelly Y, Zilanawala A, Booker C, Sacker A. Social media use and adolescent mental health: findings from the UK millennium cohort study. EClinicalMedicine. 2019;6:59–68. Published 2019 Jan 4
27. Lee DS, Jiang T, Crocker J, Way BM. Social media use and its link to physical health indicators. Cyberpsychol Behav Soc Netw. 2022;25(2):87–93. https://doi.org/10.1089/cyber.2021.0188.
28. Barile J, Margolis A, Cason G, Kim R, Kalash S, Tchaconas A, et al. Diagnostic accuracy of a large language model in pediatric case studies. JAMA Pediatr. 2024;178(3):313–5.

Chapter 9
Artificial Intelligence for Public Health

Terry Adirim

Introduction

AI, Machine Learning, and predictive analytics have a critical role in public health. During the COVID-19 pandemic, AI tools were used for a collection of activities: disease surveillance, contact tracing, automated screening, evaluation of established drugs for treatment, developing new drugs, predicting disease severity, and forecasting disease spread. The ability of machine learning algorithms to analyze vast datasets to identify disease patterns and predict outbreaks, and natural language processing to facilitate rapid processing of unstructured public health data provide clear examples of how technology can be used to improve public health outcomes [1]. Finally, these tools, as was demonstrated during the COVID-19 pandemic, promise to provide a substantial impact on a global scale [2]. This chapter discusses the use cases, benefits, and challenges of using AI in public health.

AI Applications in Public Health

Epidemiology, Infectious Disease Modeling and Disease Surveillance

The integration of artificial intelligence (AI) into epidemiology and disease surveillance has been transformative in public health, enabling more efficient detection, monitoring, and management of infectious diseases.

T. Adirim (✉)
Departments of Pediatrics and Preventive Medicine and Biostatistics,
Uniformed Services University of the Health Sciences, Bethesda, MD, USA

T. Adirim (ed.), *Digital Health, AI and Generative AI in Healthcare*,
https://doi.org/10.1007/978-3-031-83526-1_9

One example is predictive modeling for infectious disease outbreaks. It is important to note that AI models are only as good as the data on which they are trained, and often, the best models use a diverse set of data sources such as health records, social media, weather patterns, and travel data. During the COVID-19 pandemic, platforms such as BlueDot and HealthMap used natural language processing to scan news reports, airline data, and social media posts to provide early warnings of the outbreak before traditional public health organizations could respond [3, 4]. These systems used nontraditional data sources, and AI to help health authorities anticipate the disease's spread and prepare resources accordingly.

Disease Surveillance is another area that has been transformed by AI. Systems using algorithms to process data from emergency departments, clinics, and even pharmacies in real-time can detect abnormal patterns in healthcare usage that might indicate a disease outbreak. One such example is the Syndromic Surveillance System used by the Centers for Disease Control and Prevention (CDC) in the United States [5]. This system collects and analyzes clinical data, such as patient symptoms and medication sales, using AI to flag unusual spikes in data patterns associated with specific illnesses, allowing for swift public health responses.

AI also plays a crucial role in genomic epidemiology by helping to analyze pathogen genetics as a surrogate for tracking disease transmission. During Ebola and Zika outbreaks, AI processed genetic sequencing data to map the evolution of the viruses. These analyses allowed epidemiologists to understand how the diseases spread geographically and temporally, facilitating the development of targeted control measures [6]. Similarly, AI-driven genomic surveillance was vital in tracking the mutations of the SARS-CoV-2 virus during the COVID-19 pandemic, providing insights into the emergence of new variants and their potential impact on vaccine efficacy [7].

Additionally, AI-driven image recognition tools assist in diagnosing diseases that present with specific physical symptoms [8]. In the case of diseases like tuberculosis, AI algorithms analyze chest X-rays to detect abnormalities indicative of infection. Projects like CAD4TB (Computer-Aided Detection for Tuberculosis) have been deployed in resource-limited settings to support rapid screening and diagnosis, thereby aiding in timely epidemiological surveillance and intervention.

In vector-borne diseases such as malaria or dengue fever, AI-based systems utilize satellite imagery to identify potential breeding grounds by analyzing environmental factors like rainfall, temperature, and vegetation cover [9, 10]. This information allows health officials to predict disease hotspots and allocate resources for targeted interventions. For example, IBM's Watson Health partnered with public health agencies to use AI in analyzing weather and environmental data to predict outbreaks of mosquito-borne diseases, leading to more effective disease control strategies.

Overall, AI enhances the capabilities of epidemiologists by providing timely and accurate analysis of diverse datasets, facilitating early detection of outbreaks, improving resource allocation, and enabling rapid responses to emerging health threats. As AI technology continues to evolve, its role in epidemiology and disease surveillance is expected to grow, offering increasingly sophisticated methods for protecting public health.

AI Use for Disease Monitoring and Analytics

Wearable devices and smart thermometers have been used to monitor physiological data, helping to track the onset of diseases like influenza and COVID-19. These tools collect continuous data on metrics such as body temperature and heart rate, which can indicate illness before symptoms fully manifest and disease has spread [11]. This data can be aggregated and analyzed to make predictions about diseases within communities with the potential to assist public health officials in determining interventions.

Wearable devices such as smartwatches and fitness trackers have evolved with the potential to monitor a wide range of health parameters, including heart rate, blood oxygen levels (SpO2), body temperature, and sleep patterns [12]. During the COVID-19 pandemic, wearable devices such as Fitbit, Oura Ring, and the Apple Watch were utilized in research studies to detect early signs of illness. Changes in an individual's resting heart rate, respiratory rate, or sleep quality can signal the onset of an infection [13]. By aggregating data from large numbers of users, public health officials have the potential to identify potential hotspots and trends in illness prevalence within a community. For instance, studies have shown that deviations in heart rate and activity patterns recorded by wearables can correlate with flu-like symptoms, providing a means for large-scale, passive health monitoring.

Smart thermometers, such as those produced by companies like Kinsa, offer another layer of surveillance by capturing and analyzing body temperature data in real time [14]. These thermometers connect to smartphones, uploading temperature readings and associated symptoms to a centralized database. The aggregated data is then anonymized and analyzed to detect unusual increases in fever rates, which can indicate the emergence or spread of infectious diseases. During the flu season and the COVID-19 pandemic, Kinsa's network of smart thermometers provided critical early warning signs of fever spikes in specific geographic regions, offering insights into where the disease might be spreading [15].

One key benefit of using these devices for disease surveillance is the ability to collect health data continuously and at a granular level, both at the individual and community scale. The early detection of abnormal health patterns through wearable devices and smart thermometers allows health authorities to respond quickly to potential outbreaks, allocate resources more effectively, and implement targeted interventions [16]. Furthermore, these technologies empower individuals to take a proactive role in monitoring their health, contributing to the overall public health ecosystem.

The integration of wearable devices and smart thermometers into public health surveillance systems also presents opportunities for personalized health interventions. For example, individuals receiving real-time feedback about their health status can be prompted to seek medical care, self-isolate, or adjust their behavior based on symptoms. This personalized approach enhances community-wide efforts to contain the spread of infectious diseases and supports a more resilient public health infrastructure. As these technologies continue to evolve, their role in disease surveillance is expected to expand, providing increasingly sophisticated and accurate tools for monitoring and responding to health threats in communities.

Genomic Surveillance

While AI-driven disease surveillance monitors health data from multiple sources, such as healthcare facilities and social media, to predict and identify disease outbreaks, thus supporting more comprehensive public health responses, AI use in genomic surveillance focuses on analyzing the genetic sequences of pathogens to detect mutations, track disease transmission, and predict future outbreaks, playing a critical role in understanding pathogen evolution and variant emergence. Genomic sequencing provides a detailed map of a pathogen's genetic structure, which can be complex and data intensive. AI algorithms are well-suited for processing large volumes of genomic data to identify patterns and mutations in pathogens, which can significantly impact the effectiveness of treatment as pathogens evolve. During the COVID-19 pandemic, for instance, AI played a key role in analyzing millions of SARS-CoV-2 genome sequences from around the world [17, 18]. By recognizing specific genetic markers, AI helped track the emergence of variants like Delta and Omicron, offering real-time insights into how the virus evolved and spread geographically. This information allowed public health authorities to assess the impact of new variants on transmission rates, vaccine efficacy, and the severity of illness, guiding public health interventions and vaccination strategies.

In addition to mutation tracking, AI assists in phylogenetic analysis, which involves studying the evolutionary relationships between different strains of pathogens [19]. This analysis is critical in understanding how diseases spread through populations and across borders. AI models can process complex genetic data to create more accurate and faster phylogenetic trees, revealing transmission pathways that might otherwise go unnoticed. For example, during the Ebola outbreak in West Africa, AI-driven genomic surveillance helped trace the origins and spread of the virus, enabling health officials to implement targeted containment strategies. Similarly, during Zika virus outbreaks, AI was used to monitor the virus's movement and evolution, supporting efforts to predict and prevent further spread [20].

AI also enhances pathogen surveillance by automating the process of detecting antimicrobial resistance (AMR) genes within bacterial genomes. This capability is crucial in managing the growing public health threat posed by antibiotic-resistant bacteria [21]. AI algorithms analyze genomic data from bacteria isolated in clinical settings to identify resistance genes quickly, informing healthcare providers about the most effective treatments. For example, machine learning models have been developed to predict resistance patterns in tuberculosis by examining the genetic makeup of Mycobacterium tuberculosis. This has improved the speed and accuracy of diagnosis, allowing for more effective patient management, and reducing the spread of resistant strains.

Furthermore, AI-driven genomic epidemiology enables more precise outbreak forecasting. By integrating genomic data with other epidemiological information—such as patient demographics, travel history, and environmental factors—AI models can predict the trajectory of an outbreak and inform resource allocation. For example, AI has been used in the surveillance of influenza, incorporating viral genomic data and environmental factors to predict which strains are most likely to circulate in the upcoming flu season, aiding in the development of more effective vaccines [22].

In public health, AI-powered genomic surveillance is not limited to infectious diseases. It is increasingly applied to monitor the genetic changes in non-communicable diseases like cancer, aiding in understanding their progression and informing personalized treatment strategies [23]. For infectious disease surveillance, the combination of AI and genomics provides a powerful approach to early detection, rapid response, and effective disease control, ultimately enhancing global health security. As genomic sequencing technology becomes more accessible and affordable, and as AI algorithms grow more sophisticated, their integration into public health strategies promises a future of more proactive and precise disease management.

AI and Environmental Health

AI enabled systems can analyze environmental data, such as climate conditions, to predict disease outbreaks related to environmental changes. Additionally, behavioral data from mobile devices and social media can provide insights into population movements and behaviors that may influence disease spread [24, 25].

AI is increasingly used in environmental health to monitor, predict, and mitigate the effects of environmental factors on public health. By analyzing large datasets from various sources such as satellite imagery, climate data, air quality measurements, and geographic information systems (GIS), AI enables researchers and public health officials to identify patterns, detect hazards, and develop targeted interventions to protect communities from environmental risks.

One of the primary applications of AI in environmental health is air quality monitoring and prediction [26]. AI models process real-time data from air quality sensors and meteorological sources to monitor levels of pollutants like particulate matter (PM2.5 and PM10), nitrogen dioxide (NO2), sulfur dioxide (SO2), and ozone (O3) [27]. These models can then predict pollution levels based on factors such as weather patterns, traffic, and industrial activities. For example, the use of neural networks has allowed researchers to forecast air pollution episodes with high accuracy, enabling governments to issue health warnings and implement measures to reduce exposure. In cities like Beijing and Los Angeles, AI-supported air quality monitoring systems provide residents with real-time information on pollutant levels, helping individuals make informed decisions to protect their health, especially those with respiratory conditions [28].

Climate change and its impact on health is another area where AI plays a crucial role. AI is used to analyze vast amounts of climate data, such as temperature changes, precipitation patterns, and extreme weather events, to predict the occurrence of climate-related health issues. For example, AI models can identify regions at higher risk for heatwaves and predict their potential health impacts, including heat-related illnesses and deaths. These insights allow for the implementation of public health interventions, such as establishing cooling centers and issuing early warnings to vulnerable populations. AI also helps in modeling the spread of vector-borne diseases, such as malaria and dengue, which are influenced by climatic factors [29]. By integrating data on weather, vegetation, and human population movement, AI can forecast changes in the habitats of disease-carrying vectors, aiding in the development of strategies to control and prevent disease transmission.

AI's role in water quality assessment is another crucial aspect of environmental health. Traditional water testing methods can be time-consuming and costly. In contrast, AI models analyze data from remote sensors, satellite images, and historical water quality measurements to quickly assess the health of water bodies. For instance, machine learning algorithms process satellite imagery to detect harmful algal blooms (HABs) in lakes and oceans [30]. These blooms can release toxins harmful to human health and marine life. AI's ability to detect early signs of HABs enables timely interventions, such as issuing public health advisories and adjusting water treatment processes. Additionally, AI algorithms help predict contamination events in water supply systems, allowing for proactive measures to prevent the spread of waterborne diseases [31].

In the context of exposure to hazardous chemicals, AI enhances environmental health surveillance by detecting and evaluating potential chemical hazards in the environment. AI tools process large datasets containing information about chemical properties, emissions from industries, and soil and water samples to identify regions with elevated risk of chemical exposure [32]. For example, AI-driven analysis of satellite data helps identify illegal dumping of toxic waste and contamination from industrial activities, facilitating quicker responses to environmental hazards. Moreover, AI-powered toxicology models, using deep learning and natural language processing (NLP), predict the toxicity of chemicals based on their molecular structures [33]. This application accelerates the risk assessment process, supporting regulatory bodies in making informed decisions to limit exposure to harmful substances.

Overall, AI's applications in environmental health contribute to more efficient monitoring and risk management. By providing timely, accurate, and actionable information, AI helps public health officials and policymakers implement targeted interventions to mitigate environmental health risks, enhancing the overall well-being of communities. As AI technologies continue to evolve, their integration into environmental health practices promises a more proactive and data-driven approach to safeguarding public health.

AI Use Cases for Health Promotion and Disease Prevention

Artificial Intelligence (AI) can have a role in health promotion and disease prevention strategies. For public health interventions, AI has the potential to support design of targeted vaccine and screening programs. AI's capability to process vast amounts of data and predict virus mutations has significantly accelerated vaccine development timelines. For instance, during the COVID-19 pandemic, AI-driven algorithms enabled rapid identification of viral variants, facilitating the adaptation of vaccines to new strains in record time [34].

Identifying high-risk populations is another critical area where AI excels. By leveraging predictive analytics, AI algorithms analyze diverse datasets encompassing demographic, genetic, and environmental factors to identify individuals at heightened risk of developing specific diseases. For example, predictive models can forecast cardiovascular risks based on lifestyle factors and genetic predispositions, enabling healthcare providers to implement targeted interventions such as lifestyle modifications and early medical interventions [35]. Such precision in risk assessment enables healthcare systems to allocate resources more efficiently, focusing preventive measures where they are most needed, thereby mitigating disease burdens within communities.

In addition to targeted interventions, AI enhances health education and communication efforts through innovations like virtual assistants and chatbots. These AI-driven tools provide personalized health information and support to individuals, promoting health literacy and empowering patients to manage their health effectively. Virtual assistants equipped with natural language processing (NLP) capabilities can interact conversationally with users, offering real-time guidance on health-related queries and delivering tailored educational content [36]. This capability not only improves access to healthcare information but also facilitates patient engagement and adherence to preventive health practices.

AI-Driven Targeted Population Health Prevention Strategies

AI applications have the potential to drive targeted prevention strategies in population health by identifying at-risk individuals and groups, predicting future health risks, and designing personalized interventions. By analyzing large-scale datasets, including electronic health records (EHRs), social determinants of health (SDOH), genetic information, and behavioral data, AI can uncover patterns and risk factors that traditional methods might miss. For example, machine learning algorithms can analyze community data to identify populations at high risk for conditions like diabetes or cardiovascular disease [37]. Kaiser Permanente used AI to identify patients at risk of developing Type 2 diabetes by examining factors such as BMI, blood pressure, and family history [38]. The system flagged high-risk patients, allowing healthcare providers to offer targeted lifestyle modifications, nutrition counseling, and exercise programs tailored to individual needs, effectively reducing the incidence of diabetes in the identified population. Similarly, in the realm of cardiovascular health, AI models have been used to predict heart attack risks in individuals by analyzing EHRs for indicators like cholesterol levels, smoking status, and past medical history, facilitating early interventions through medication and lifestyle adjustments [39].

Additionally, AI supports the design and implementation of precision public health campaigns. For example, AI has been used in targeting mental health interventions in communities. In a project by the University of Washington, researchers used AI to analyze electronic health records and social determinants data to identify individuals potentially at high risk of suicide [40]. The AI inputs included factors such as past mental health conditions, medication history, socioeconomic status, and patterns of healthcare utilization. Based on the AI's predictions, mental health providers were able to offer early and targeted interventions, such as counseling, therapy, and social support services, tailored to those most at risk [41]. Similarly, AI models have been applied to identify neighborhoods with high rates of opioid overdoses [42]. By analyzing data on prescription patterns, emergency response reports, and socioeconomic factors, AI helped public health authorities implement targeted outreach programs, including distributing naloxone kits and providing community education on substance use [43]. These targeted strategies, informed by AI, enable more efficient resource allocation and more effective preventive measures, ultimately reducing the health burden in vulnerable populations.

Behavioral Modification AI Applications

Challenges of AI for Public Health

Despite advancements, integrating AI into public health systems poses significant challenges. Ethical considerations surrounding data privacy and consent are critical considerations, particularly as AI relies on extensive personal health data for its predictive capabilities. The effectiveness of AI systems depends on the accuracy, quality, and comprehensiveness of the data analyzed [44]. Ensuring transparency and fairness in AI algorithms is crucial to prevent biases and maintain trust among diverse populations. Recognizing and addressing biases in public health data on which AI driven population tools are based cannot be emphasized enough and is critical to ensuring trust in vulnerable communities. Transparent practices and inclusive policies are essential to address these issues and maintain public trust [45]. Furthermore, healthcare professionals require adequate training to effectively utilize AI tools and interpret their outputs accurately. Bridging these knowledge gaps is essential for maximizing the potential of AI in augmenting public health initiatives and optimizing patient outcomes.

Robust data governance frameworks are necessary to protect sensitive health information. Integrating AI systems with existing public health infrastructure can be challenging. Ensuring that different systems and datasets can work together seamlessly is crucial for maximizing the benefits of AI in disease surveillance. Implementing AI solutions requires significant technological infrastructure and expertise, which may be lacking in low-resource settings. Investments in technology and capacity building are needed to ensure equitable access to AI-driven health solutions.

Summary

AI in public health has the potential to transform public health by predicting pandemics, monitoring diseases in real time and promoting targeted health interventions. Future efforts for incorporating AI into public health should focus on addressing the challenges of data integration and ethical considerations, ensuring that AI technologies are implemented in a manner that is both effective and equitable. As AI continues to evolve, its role in disease surveillance will undoubtedly expand, offering new opportunities to safeguard public health.

References

1. Hamilton AJ, Strauss AT, Martinez DA, Hinson JS, Levin S, Lin G, Klein EY. Machine learning and artificial intelligence: applications in healthcare epidemiology. Antimicrob Steward Healthc Epidemiol. 2021;1(1):e28. Published October 7, 2021.
2. Olawade DB, Wada OJ, David-Olawade AC, Kunonga E, Abaire O, Ling J. Using artificial intelligence to improve public health: a narrative review. Front. Public Health. 2023;11:1196397. Published October 26, 2023.
3. Bogoch II, Watts A, Thomas-Bachli A, et al. Pneumonia of unknown etiology in Wuhan, China: potential for international spread via commercial air travel. J Travel Med. 2020;27(2):taaa008.
4. Brownstein JS, Freifeld CC, Reis BY, Mandl KD. Surveillance Sans Frontières: internet-based emerging infectious disease intelligence and the HealthMap project. PLoS Med. 2008;5(7):e151.
5. Centers for Disease Control and Prevention (CDC). National Syndromic Surveillance Program (NSSP): enhancing public health surveillance. Published 2021. https://www.cdc.gov/nssp/. Accessed 15 Sept 2024.
6. Gardy JL, Loman NJ. Towards a genomics-informed, real-time, global pathogen surveillance system. Nat Rev Genet. 2018;19(1):9–20.
7. Shu Y, McCauley J. GISAID: Global initiative on sharing all influenza data—from vision to reality. EuroSurveillance. 2017;22(13):30494.
8. Qin ZZ, Sander MS, Rai B, Titahong CN, Sudrungrot S, Laah SN, et al. Using artificial intelligence to read chest radiographs for tuberculosis detection: a multi-site evaluation of the diagnostic accuracy of three deep learning systems. Sci Rep. 2019;9(1):1–10.
9. Akhtar M, Kraemer MUG, Gardner LM. A dynamic neural network model for predicting risk of Zika in real time. BMC Med. 2019;17:171.
10. Anno S, Hara T, Kai H, et al. Spatiotemporal dengue fever hotspots associated with climatic factors in Taiwan including outbreak predictions based on machine-learning. Geospat Health. 2019;14(2). https://doi.org/10.4081/gh.2019.771.

11. Best J. Wearable technology: covid-19 and the rise of remote clinical monitoring. BMJ. 2021;372:n413. Published 2021 Feb 18.
12. Mishra T, Wang M, Metwally AA, Bogu GK, Brooks AW, Bahmani A, et al. Pre-symptomatic detection of COVID-19 from smartwatch data. Nat Biomed Eng. 2020;4:1208–20.
13. Quer G, Radin JM, Gadaleta M, Baca-Motes K, Ariniello L, Ramos E, et al. Wearable sensor data and self-reported symptoms for COVID-19 detection. Nat Med. 2021;27:73–7.
14. Kinsa Health. Kinsa's early warning identification and management capabilities. https://home.kinsahealth.com/research/kinsa-early-warning-technical-summary. Accessed 16 Sept 2024.
15. Miller AC, Foti NJ, Lewnard JA, Jewell NP, Guestrin C. Deploying an early warning system for influenza-like illness using wearable devices and smart thermometers. Epidemiol Infect. 2020;148
16. Jain S, Bansal R, Sikarwar B. Smart wearables: novel strategies for the early detection of infectious diseases. J Infect Public Health. 2021;14(8):1075–81.
17. Meredith LW, Hamilton WL, Warne B, Houldcroft CJ, Hosmillo M, Jahun AS, et al. Rapid implementation of SARS-CoV-2 sequencing to investigate cases of health-care associated COVID-19: a prospective genomic surveillance study. Lancet Infect Dis. 2020;20(11):1263–72.
18. Viana R, Moyo S, Amoako DG, Tegally H, Scheepers C, Althaus CL, et al. Rapid epidemic expansion of the SARS-CoV-2 Omicron variant in southern Africa. Nature. 2022;603(7902):679–86.
19. Dudas G, Carvalho LM, Bedford T, Tatem AJ, Baele G, Faria NR, et al. Virus genomes reveal factors that spread and sustained the Ebola epidemic. Nature. 2017;544(7650):309–15.
20. Grubaugh ND, Ladner JT, Kraemer MU, Dudas G, Tan AL, Gangavarapu K, et al. Genomic epidemiology reveals multiple introductions of Zika virus into the United States. Nature. 2017;546(7658):401–5.
21. Yang Y, Niehaus KE, Walker TM, Iqbal Z, Walker AS, Wilson DJ, et al. Machine learning for classifying tuberculosis drug-resistance from DNA sequencing data. Bioinformatics. 2018;34(10):1666–71.
22. Bedford T, Riley S, Barr IG, Broor S, Chadha M, Cox NJ, et al. Global circulation patterns of seasonal influenza viruses vary with antigenic drift. Nature. 2015;523(7559):217–20. https://doi.org/10.1038/nature14460.
23. Frasca M, La Torre D, Repetto M, De Nicolò V, Pravettoni G, Cutica I. Artificial intelligence applications to genomic data in cancer research: a review of recent trends and emerging areas. Discov Anal. 2024;2:10.
24. Wilson AE, Lehmann CU, Saleh SN, Hanna J, Medford RJ. Social media: a new tool for outbreak surveillance. Antimicrob Steward Healthc Epidemiol. 2021;1(1):e50.
25. Kostkova P, Saigi-Rubio F, Eguia H, Borbolla D, Verschuuren M, Hamilton C, et al. Data and digital solutions to support surveillance strategies in the context of the COVID-19 pandemic. Front Digit Health. 2021;3:707902.
26. Wei J, Li Z, Lyapustin A, et al. A high-resolution data-driven estimate of global surface ozone concentrations. Environ Sci Technol Lett. 2020;7(11):828–34.
27. Schneider P, Dinterman PA. Assessing urban air quality using real-time data and machine learning. Environ Monit Assess. 2019;191(6):347.
28. Wu X, Lu Y, Zhou S, Chen L, Xu B. Impact of climate change on human infectious diseases: empirical evidence and human adaptation. Environ Int. 2016;86:14–23.
29. Ryan SJ, Carlson CJ, Mordecai EA, Johnson LR. Global expansion and redistribution of Aedes-borne virus transmission risk with climate change. PLoS Negl Trop Dis. 2019;13(3):e0007213.
30. Kriebel M, Peter L. AI-based detection of harmful algal blooms from remote sensing imagery in freshwater lakes. Remote Sens Environ. 2021;263:112542.
31. Reed PM, Kasprzyk JR. Water quality assessment and prediction using data-driven models and machine learning techniques. J Environ Manag. 2009;90(3):2076–88.
32. Zhang C, Wang H, Ji Y, Wang Q, Su Y. Machine learning-based toxicity prediction: an overview of the state-of-the-art and future prospects. Chemosphere. 2019;227:441–8.
33. Marvuglia A, Benetto E, Rege S, Jury C. AI-enabled satellite remote sensing for monitoring of hazardous waste sites. Sci Total Environ. 2020;728:138618.

34. Smith A, Jones B, et al. AI-driven strategies for rapid vaccine development: case studies from the COVID-19 pandemic. J Public Health Technol. 2021;25(2):112–25.
35. Brown E, Li H, et al. Predictive analytics and AI in cardiovascular risk assessment: applications and implications for public health. J Health Anal. 2019;12(1):56–68.
36. Li J, Smith R, et al. Virtual assistants and chatbots in healthcare: enhancing patient engagement and health literacy. J Med Commun. 2021;30(3):198–210.
37. Tomar D, Agarwal S. A comparison of various optimization algorithms in developing a model for type 2 diabetes risk prediction. Comput Biol Med. 2016;76:52–61.
38. Montori VM, Ismail-Beigi F. The unfulfilled promise of individualized care in diabetes. JAMA. 2020;324(8):731–2.
39. Krittanawong C, Zhang H, Wang Z, Aydar M, Kitai T. Artificial intelligence in precision cardiovascular medicine. J Am Coll Cardiol. 2017;69(21):2657–64.
40. Boudreaux ED, McCabe B, Soberay KA. Machine learning applications for suicide risk prediction. J Affect Disord. 2022;299:1–11.
41. Barak-Corren Y, Castro VM, Javitt S, et al. Predicting suicidal behavior from longitudinal electronic health records. Am J Psychiatr. 2017;174(2):154–62.
42. Hsu DJ, McCarthy ML, Stevens RD, Masurkar A. Artificial intelligence and predictive analytics for safe opioid prescribing: a review. Anesth Analg. 2021;132(5):1417–25.
43. Johnson K, Bonaventura E, Shao Y. Data analytics for enhancing opioid epidemic surveillance and community health interventions. Drug Alcohol Depend. 2020;215:108204.
44. Topol EJ. High-performance medicine: the convergence of human and artificial intelligence. Nat Med. 2019;25(1):44–56.
45. Bothra A, Cao Y, Černý J, Arora G. The epidemiology of infectious diseases meets AI: a match made in heaven. Pathogens. 2023;12(2):317.

Part III
Responsible Use of AI in Healthcare

Chapter 10
Responsible Use of AI: Ethics, Biases, and Fairness

Karen Blades

Introduction

Adoption of AI healthcare solutions come with the imperative to address the ethical challenges of AI technology, namely bias. Bias, whether gender, racial, or socioeconomic, occur due to the existing biases within the underlying data and algorithms upon which AI systems rely. Data sets upon which AI technologies are trained and built upon can be limited to one population over another overlooking entire groups of people with the potential for dire consequences. A notable example includes AI bias in the Correctional Offender Management Profiling for Alternative Sanctions (COMPRAS) tool, an algorithm used by US court systems to predict the likelihood that defendants would become recidivist. Due to the biased data that was used, the model that was chosen, and the process for creating the algorithm, the model predicted twice as many false positives for recidivism for Black offenders, 45% vs. 23% for White offenders [1]. Another example, more relevant for healthcare includes a 2019 study that found that an algorithm used to guide healthcare decisions for more than 200 million people in US hospitals predicted that White patients would likely require more medical care than Black patients. The study found racial bias reduced the number of Black patients identified for additional care by more than half because the algorithm used health costs as a proxy for healthcare needs. The study found that less money is spent on Black patients who have the same level of need as White patients, and therefore the algorithm falsely concluded that Black patients are healthier than White patients [2]. This chapter discusses biases as the top ethical challenge with AI use in healthcare and will provide recommendations to overcome the limitations of bias introduced by AI technologies.

K. Blades (✉)
WhirlyBee Consulting, Washington, DC, USA
e-mail: karen@whirlybee.com

T. Adirim (ed.), *Digital Health, AI and Generative AI in Healthcare*,
https://doi.org/10.1007/978-3-031-83526-1_10

At the end of this chapter, clinicians will be aware of:

- Ethical Principles of Healthcare AI,
- Issues of Bias, Fairness, and Transparency,
- How AI Inherits and Amplifies Human Biases,
- Case Studies of Biases in Healthcare AI, and
- Ways to Overcome the Limitations of Ethical Use of AI.

Ethical Principles of Healthcare AI

Understanding and adhering to the foundational ethical principles of healthcare is crucial for clinicians who utilize AI technologies. As digital healthcare and AI usher in a new era for healthcare, the primary principles—beneficence and non-maleficence—remain unchanged. Let's explore these principles in the context of AI, ensuring that its deployment in healthcare aligns with ethical standards [3].

Beneficence—The Principle of Doing Good

Beneficence, the ethical obligation to act for the benefit of others, is a cornerstone of healthcare. In digital health and AI, beneficence translates to leveraging these technologies to enhance patient care, improve health outcomes, and contribute to the well-being of individuals and communities.

AI technologies promise to significantly enhance patient care by equipping clinicians with advanced tools for diagnosis, treatment planning, and monitoring. Early solutions demonstrate how AI algorithms can analyze vast amounts of medical data to identify patterns and predict disease progression, leading to earlier and more accurate diagnoses. AI-powered decision support systems offer personalized treatment recommendations based on the latest evidence and patient-specific factors, optimizing care delivery. Additionally, AI enhances patient monitoring through wearable devices and remote health monitoring systems, providing real-time insights into a patient's condition, and enabling timely interventions.

By augmenting the capabilities of healthcare professionals, AI can lead to more effective, efficient, and personalized care, ultimately promoting patients' well-being and contributing to the patient's best overall interests.

Non-maleficence—The Principle of Not Harming Patients

Non-maleficence, the obligation to "do no harm," is foundational to medical ethics. Just as AI promises to revolutionize healthcare, it also poses significant risks that clinicians must identify and carefully manage to prevent harm to patients. Many of these harms, like bias, are not initially evident.

The main concern with AI in healthcare is the potential for errors or biases in AI algorithms, which can lead to incorrect diagnoses, inappropriate treatment recommendations, and adverse patient outcomes. AI systems are only as good as the datasets on which they are trained. If the training data is biased or incomplete, then the AI's outputs will also be flawed, perpetuating existing disparities in healthcare.

Furthermore, the complexity and allure of AI algorithms presents obstacles for clinicians in understanding and trusting AI-generated recommendations, potentially leading to either overreliance on AI or skepticism that undermines its benefits. Ensuring the safety and reliability of AI adoption requires rigorous testing, validation, continuous monitoring, and transparent communication about the limitations and uncertainties associated with AI-driven decisions.

Some areas at risk include challenges to patient autonomy, consent, and privacy concerns with patient health data, fair access, and equitable health outcomes, and ensuring fair access to AI technologies. Let's examine each of these risks.

Challenges to Patient Autonomy Patient autonomy, the right to make informed healthcare decisions, is a fundamental ethical principle. The use of AI systems can both enhance and challenge patient autonomy, particularly in areas related to consent and privacy.

Consent and Privacy Concerns AI systems require access to large amounts of personal health data to function effectively. Ensuring that patients provide informed consent for using their data is vital. Still, the complexity of AI technologies can make it difficult for patients to fully understand how their data will be used and the potential risks involved. Transparent communication and robust consent processes are necessary to uphold patient autonomy.

Privacy concerns also arise with using AI in healthcare. The vast amount of data required for AI systems increases the risk of data breaches and unauthorized access to sensitive health information. Ensuring compliance with privacy regulations while implementing strong data security measures is crucial to protect patient autonomy and maintain trust in AI technologies. See Chap. 12 for more on Data Privacy and Security.

Fair Access and Equitable Health Outcomes The principle of justice in healthcare emphasizes the fair distribution of resources and equitable access to care. AI technologies, depending on how they are implemented and accessed, have the potential to either mitigate or exacerbate health disparities.

Ensuring Fair Access to AI Technologies It is essential to ensure that AI technologies are accessible to all patients, regardless of socioeconomic status, geographic location, or other factors. Ensuring fair access includes addressing barriers to access, such as the cost of AI-powered tools and digital or technology deserts that prevent certain populations from benefiting from AI advancements.

Moreover, AI systems must be designed and trained to provide equitable health outcomes across diverse patient populations. Equitable outcomes require using diverse and representative data in AI training processes to avoid biases that could lead to unequal treatment recommendations and health outcomes. Continuous evaluation and refinement of AI systems are necessary to ensure they promote fairness and justice in healthcare.

By understanding and applying these ethical principles, clinicians will be equipped to navigate the complexities of AI in healthcare effectively. They will recognize AI's potential to enhance patient care while being aware of its limitations and risks. Advocating for rigorous testing and validation of AI systems will be crucial to ensuring patient safety and minimizing harm. Clinicians will also uphold patient autonomy by prioritizing transparent communication, informed consent, and robust data privacy protections. Furthermore, they will strive for justice by promoting fair access to AI technologies and ensuring equitable health outcomes for all patients.

Adherence to these ethical principles will guide the responsible and effective use of AI in healthcare, ultimately improving patient care and advancing the field of digital health.

Bias, Fairness, and Transparency in AI Models

While AI is poised to transform healthcare, it is necessary to address the issues of bias, fairness, and transparency that will impact the effectiveness and ethical use of AI technologies. What exactly is considered bias? What are the challenges and implications of bias? What are the mitigation strategies for bias? Answering these questions will give clinicians the knowledge to prepare to leverage AI technologies ethically and effectively, contributing to improved and equitable healthcare outcomes.

Types of Biases and Their Origins

Bias in AI models or systems can arise from various sources and significantly affect the accuracy and fairness of AI-driven healthcare solutions. The two primary types of biases are data bias and algorithmic bias [4].

Data bias occurs when the datasets used to train the AI model or system are unrepresentative or imbalanced, leading to skewed outcomes. Data bias can result from data sets containing historical healthcare access, treatment, and clinical research inequalities. Underrepresenting certain demographic groups in medical datasets can lead to AI models performing poorly for those populations. A noteworthy issue is the underrepresentation of women, African Americans, and Latinos in healthcare datasets derived from clinical research. Although the adoption of public laws like the NIH Revitalization Act of 1993 seeks to address the lack of gender and ethnic diversity in clinical research data, most training datasets for healthcare AI

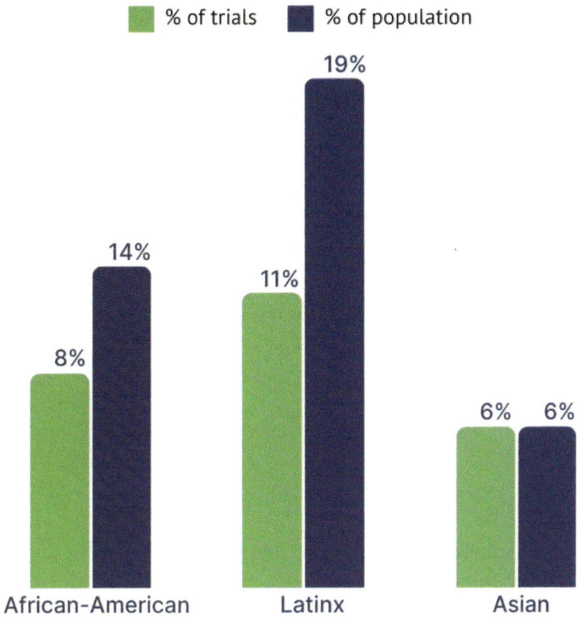

Fig. 10.1 A recent analysis of 32,000 participants in new drug trials in the U.S. in 2020 shows that African Americans and Latinos are significantly underrepresented in clinical trials compared to their representation in the overall population [7, 8]

technologies continue to base diagnostic tools and treatment recommendations on data from clinical trials where 86% of participants are white and usually male producing tools that are less accurate for women, African-Americans, or Latinos, perpetuating existing health disparities [5, 6] (Fig. 10.1).

Lack of diversity in clinical trials can lead to the development of drugs that only work for some people—or may even harm whole segments of the population. It also creates research conditions that ignore diverse genetic, environmental, cultural, and lifestyle factors that play a vital role in the development and treatment of medical conditions. Everyone must be represented for medical research to work properly [5, 11] (Fig. 10.2).

Algorithmic bias occurs when algorithms make decisions that systematically disadvantage certain groups of people. This bias is often due to the assumptions and decisions made during the development of the AI system. Developers can unintentionally introduce these biases, which may reflect broader societal biases. For instance, if an algorithm omits the specific needs of diverse populations, it may favor certain groups over others, leading to inequitable healthcare outcomes like those seen in the algorithm used to guide healthcare decisions for more than 200 million people in US hospitals which falsely predicted that White patients would likely need more medical care than Black patients for the similar medical conditions [12].

The impact of data and algorithmic bias can also be extended through clinical data and practices that make use of race correction and perpetuate or even amplify race-based health inequities [13].

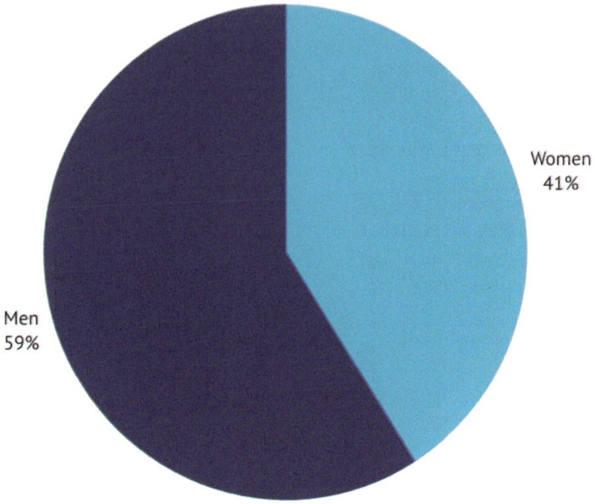

Fig. 10.2 While progress has been made, data from 2016 to 2020 show that women still only make up 40–42% of major clinical trials for cardiac, cancer, and psychiatric diseases despite comprising a higher number of patients for those diseases [9, 10]

Ensuring fairness in the use of AI systems by clinicians is integral to providing equitable healthcare. Fairness in AI means that the data models, algorithms, and AI policies or frameworks should perform equally well across different demographic groups and not systematically disadvantage any particular group. To promote fairness within their adopted AI systems, healthcare organizations and clinicians will need to apply practical methods to measure fairness, such as:

1. ***Regular audits for bias*** across diverse datasets to identify and address any disparities in outcomes.
2. ***Develop fairness metrics*** on demographic parity, equal opportunity, and disparate impact to evaluate and compare the performance of AI models across different groups.
3. Ensure ***inclusive data collection*** is representative of the population served to mitigate data bias and improve fairness.
4. Request ***algorithmic adjustments*** as you gather new data from re-sampling and establish fairness-aware algorithms to reduce bias.

As crucial as establishing fair measurement methods is, ensuring transparency in AI systems' methodologies, data sources, and decision-making processes is equally important for clinicians, patients, and regulatory bodies. Such transparency fosters trust and accountability by allowing for the identification and correction of bias in the AI system. It also supports informed consent by enabling patients to understand how their data will be used and the implications of AI-driven decisions. Additionally, transparency helps ensure regulatory compliance with legal and ethical standards, including data protection regulations and medical ethics guidelines.

By addressing the critical issues of bias, fairness, and transparency in healthcare AI models and systems, clinicians will recognize different types of biases by understanding the origins and implications of data and algorithmic bias in AI, mainly as they affect underrepresented groups in healthcare. They will also promote fair AI systems by advocating for and implementing methods to measure and enhance the fairness of AI technologies, ensuring equitable health outcomes for all patients. Lastly, emphasize the importance of transparency in AI methodologies and decision-making processes, fostering trust and accountability in AI-driven healthcare.

AI Inherits and Amplifies Human Biases

While powerful and innovative, AI systems are not immune to the biases present in human society. Healthcare has its share of bias inherited from historical research, like race correction. Race correction refers to using race to influence how a patient is treated. One example is the bias built into spirometer calculations that often apply a race correction based on a nineteenth-century research study using the false premise that African Americans have lower lung capacity. Data from this research exacerbated disparities during the COVID-19 pandemic [14–16].

The data or tool does not have to be race-corrected to inherit human bias. Pulse oximetry, a common tool in healthcare that relies on software algorithms, while not a tool that has been race-corrected, created problems during the COVID-19 pandemic because pulse oximeters are notoriously inaccurate for people with dark skin. These inaccuracies resulted in Black patients, receiving intensive care, having more than a two-fold higher probability of falsely higher pulse oximetry readings compared to White patients receiving intensive care, a bias that risked undertreating this population. Most studies in the 1990s and 2000s reaffirmed those concerns in various clinical settings [17].

As introduced in Types of Bias above, these biases integrate into AI systems via the bias in the dataset or the algorithmic design. The potential to amplify these biases leads to significant ethical and practical challenges in healthcare. Clinicians need to be acutely aware of data and algorithmic bias since these biases have a considerable impact on the accuracy and fairness of AI-driven healthcare solutions.

Integration of Biases into AI Systems

The data used to train AI systems often reflects the biases present in the society from which it is collected. If the training data is biased or unrepresentative, the AI model will learn and perpetuate those biases via historical data or sampling bias (Table 10.1).

Algorithms embedded with bias can lead to clinicians misdiagnosing medical conditions or delaying critical treatment. Algorithmic biases emerge from the design choices of AI developers, which guide the AI system's feature selection and objective functions [13] (Table 10.2).

Table 10.1 Historical data and sampling bias

Historical data	Sampling bias
Medical records and historically collected health data may reflect past healthcare access and treatment disparities. The AI model will inherit these biases if these biased datasets are used without adjustment. While yet to be verified, historical data may contribute to how computers, without clinical data, know if a chest X-ray belongs to a white or black patient. If the Al system can tell if a patient is black or white, rich or poor, binary or non-binary, then the system will use that information to make decisions [18, 19].	If certain groups are underrepresented in the training data, the AI system may not perform well for these populations. Underrepresentation can stem from socioeconomic factors, geographical disparities, or historical neglect of specific communities in healthcare research. The lack of diversity in clinical trials underscores how this underrepresentation can lead to the development of drugs that only work for some people—or may even harm whole segments of the population [20, 21].

Table 10.2 Features and objective functions

Feature selection	Objective functions
Deciding which variables or features to include in the model can introduce bias. If relevant features that capture the nuances of diverse populations left out, the model may favor certain groups over others.	The goals and metrics used to optimize the AI model can embed biases. For example, an algorithm optimized solely for accuracy might perform well on the majority population but poorly on minority groups, leading to unequal treatment recommendations. This bias is often seen in medical devices and highlighted during the COVID-19 pandemic when infrared thermometer readings were impaired for people of color [14].

AI systems can not only inherit biases from data and design but also amplify them in their outputs. Consider the examples of diagnostic tools and predictive analytics to examine how AI can exacerbate existing inequalities:

Amplification Example 1: Diagnostic Tools

AI diagnostic tools trained on predominantly white populations may fail to diagnose conditions in African American or Latino patients accurately. Suppose the diagnostic tool was meant to detect skin conditions and primarily trained on images of lighter skin. In that case, the tool might be less effective for darker skin tones, leading to misdiagnosis or delayed treatment for minority patients, worsening health disparities [3].

Amplification Example 1: Predictive Analytics

Predictive analytics tools that allocate healthcare resources may disadvantage minority groups if the underlying data reflects historical biases. For example, an AI system predicting hospital readmissions might disproportionately flag minority patients as high-risk due to correlations with socioeconomic factors, leading to increased surveillance and unnecessary interventions for these patients.

By understanding the processes through which AI inherits and amplifies biases, clinicians will be able to recognize mechanisms of bias integration and gain insight into how biases get into AI systems through data and algorithm design choices. They will also understand the consequences of bias amplification. They will be aware of real-world examples of AI amplifying biases and the significant ethical and practical consequences of such amplifications. Lastly, clinicians can support the mitigation of biases in AI and understand the importance of recognizing and addressing biases in AI systems to ensure more equitable healthcare outcomes.

Understanding these biases helps clinicians critically evaluate their AI tools, ensuring that their recommendations and decisions are equitable and accurate for all patient populations. Awareness of data bias allows clinicians to advocate for more diverse and representative data sets while understanding how algorithmic bias enables them to identify and challenge potentially harmful design choices in AI systems. This knowledge helps clinicians avoid perpetuating existing health disparities, ensures better patient outcomes, and fosters trust in AI technologies.

Case Studies/Examples of Biases in Healthcare AI

Examining real-world examples of biases in healthcare AI illustrates the tangible impact of these issues when adopting AI and highlights the necessity of addressing them. This section presents three case studies that showcase racial, gender, and socioeconomic biases in AI applications within the healthcare sector.

Case Study 1: Racial Bias in Diagnostic Algorithms

United Healthcare Algorithm One of the most notable examples of racial bias in healthcare AI is algorithmic bias, which involves an algorithm developed by United Healthcare's subsidiary, Optum. The algorithm was designed to predict which patients would benefit most from additional healthcare support. However, health systems using the algorithm discovered it exhibited significant racial bias [2, 22].

The algorithm used healthcare costs as a proxy for health needs, assuming higher healthcare costs correlated with more significant health needs. However, because African American patients historically received less healthcare than their white counterparts, their healthcare costs were lower. As a result, the algorithm underestimated the health needs of African American patients compared to white patients with similar health conditions.

This algorithmic bias led to African American patients being less likely to be identified for additional healthcare support, perpetuating existing disparities in healthcare access and outcomes. The case underscores the critical need for developing AI models that consider the underlying social determinants of health and be trained on data that accurately reflects the needs of diverse populations.

The use of this diagnostic algorithm has led to a class action lawsuit alleging that United Health used the algorithm to "prematurely and in bad faith" halt payments for healthcare services. The lawsuit has yet to be resolved at the time of this publication [23].

Case Study 2: Gender Disparities in Treatment Recommendations

Cardiovascular Disease Diagnosis AI systems used in diagnosing cardiovascular diseases have shown gender disparities in their recommendations. Historically, medical research and clinical trials have predominantly included male participants, making diagnostic criteria and treatment guidelines more suited to male patients.

An AI tool designed to predict the risk of heart attacks may use symptom profiles and biomarkers that are more typical in men. However, women often present atypical symptoms for cardiovascular diseases compared to men, such as nausea or fatigue, which were less frequently recognized by such AI tools. This discrepancy can lead to underdiagnosis or delayed diagnosis and undertreatment of cardiovascular diseases in women. Due to this male default, women are 50% more likely to receive a wrong diagnosis after a heart attack [24, 25].

Consequences Women experience delays in receiving appropriate care for cardiovascular issues, leading to worse health outcomes. This case highlights the importance of including diverse patient data in AI training sets and developing gender-sensitive diagnostic tools.

Case Study 3: Socioeconomic Bias in Health Resource Distribution

Allocation of Preventive Care Resources Socioeconomic bias in AI can affect the distribution of healthcare resources. AI solutions that allocate preventive care resources, such as vaccines or screening programs, may inadvertently favor wealthier populations if they rely on data correlating healthcare utilization with socioeconomic status [26].

An AI model predicting which areas would benefit most from a new screening program might prioritize neighborhoods with higher healthcare utilization rates. However, these areas are often wealthier and have better access to healthcare services. Conversely, lower-income areas with historically lower healthcare utilization may not be prioritized despite potentially having higher unmet health needs.

Socioeconomic bias within AI exacerbates healthcare inequalities, usually with poorer communities receiving fewer resources and preventive care interventions. To counteract this, AI models should incorporate measures of healthcare needs that go beyond utilization rates, such as social determinants of health and community health indicators. These case studies offer a view into the impact of AI healthcare solutions with underlying bias built within the data or algorithm. Through these examples, clinicians will gain a nuanced understanding of how biases manifest in AI applications, revealing their real-world implications. They will recognize the profound impact of such biases, which can lead to underdiagnosis, unequal treatment, and misallocation of resources, thereby exacerbating health disparities. Armed with this knowledge, clinicians will be better equipped to advocate for improved AI practices, promoting more inclusive and representative data in AI training and developing algorithms that address the diverse needs of all patient populations.

These insights will help clinicians critically evaluate AI tools, contribute to more equitable healthcare practices, and support the development of AI technologies that better serve all patients.

Overcoming Limitations to Ethical Use of AI

Implementing comprehensive strategies and frameworks is essential to ensuring clinicians have the processes and tools necessary for the ethical use of AI in healthcare and mitigating the biases that can arise in AI systems. Practical approaches to reducing bias include introducing ethical frameworks and emphasizing the importance of multidisciplinary collaboration.

Reducing bias in AI models and systems requires deliberate actions and efforts at various stages of the development and deployment process. For development, clinicians should serve as advisors to AI vendors to advocate for and support inclusive datasets and algorithms (Table 10.3).

The following are some key mitigation strategies for the pivotal areas of data collection and algorithmic adjustment.

Adhering to ethical frameworks and guidelines is essential for the responsible deployment of AI in healthcare. Some well-established frameworks include:

- Principles for Ethical AI: These principles typically include fairness, accountability, transparency, and privacy. Ensuring your AI systems align with these principles helps mitigate biases and promotes trust in AI technologies.

Table 10.3 Mitigation strategies

Diverse Data Collection	1. Inclusive Data Sets: Ensuring that training data is representative of the diverse populations served by healthcare systems is crucial. This involves collecting data from different demographic groups, including various ages, genders, ethnicities, and socioeconomic backgrounds. Efforts should include historically underrepresented groups to avoid perpetuating existing biases.
	2. Data Augmentation: Techniques such as data augmentation can help address imbalances in training data. By artificially increasing the representation of minority groups through techniques like oversampling, AI models can be trained to perform more equitably across different populations.
Algorithmic Adjustments	1. Fairness-Aware Algorithms: Developing and using algorithms designed to be fairness-aware can help mitigate biases. These algorithms incorporate fairness constraints during the training process to ensure that the model's performance is balanced across different demographic groups.
	2. Ask for Bias Audits and Regular Evaluation: Regularly auditing AI models for bias and evaluating their performance on diverse data sets can help identify and correct biases. This process should be continuous, with updates and adjustments made as new data becomes available.
	3. Interpretable Models: Using interpretable AI models that clearly explain their decisions can help identify and address biases. Clinicians and developers can then adjust the models based on these insights to ensure fairer outcomes.

- Ethical AI Guidelines by Professional Bodies: Organizations like the American Medical Association (AMA), the World Health Organization (WHO), and, most recently, the National Academy of Medicines' Code of Conduct for AI in Healthcare provide guidelines for the ethical use of AI in healthcare. These guidelines offer practical recommendations for clinicians and developers to follow [27–29].
- Regulatory Compliance: Adhering to regulations such as the General Data Protection Regulation (GDPR) in the European Union and the Health Insurance Portability and Accountability Act (HIPAA) in the United States ensures that AI systems respect patient privacy and data protection requirements [30, 31]. See Chap. 14 for more on AI regulatory frameworks.

Addressing biases in AI requires collaboration among various stakeholders, including ethicists, technologists, clinicians, and patients. Some collaborative approaches include:

- **Interdisciplinary Teams:** Forming interdisciplinary teams that include experts in ethics, AI technology, clinical practice, and patient advocacy can help identify and address biases from multiple perspectives. These teams can work together to develop and implement fair and ethical AI systems.
- **Stakeholder Engagement:** Engaging with patients and community representatives in exploring and adopting AI processes or systems ensures that diverse perspectives are considered. Stakeholder involvement also helps identify potential biases and areas of concern early in the selection cycle.

- **Continuous Education and Training:** Providing ongoing education and training for clinicians, AI developers, and other stakeholders on the ethical implications of AI and bias mitigation strategies is essential. This education helps build awareness and equips professionals with the knowledge to develop and use AI ethically.

Clinicians can implement a range of practical strategies to promote and maintain the ethical use of AI. By adopting these approaches, clinicians will develop bias-resilient AI systems through diverse data collection methods and fairness-aware algorithms, ensuring equitable performance across different populations. They will also adhere to established ethical standards and guidelines supporting the responsible and transparent use of AI technologies. Additionally, fostering multidisciplinary collaboration will allow clinicians to work with various stakeholders to identify and address biases, thereby ensuring that AI systems serve all patients fairly and effectively.

These practical strategies will empower clinicians to counteract AI biases and promote the ethical use of AI in healthcare, ultimately leading to more equitable and trustworthy healthcare outcomes.

Ethical Principles of Healthcare AI

The principles of beneficence, non-maleficence, autonomy, and justice are critical requirements for AI to enhance patient care, avoid harm, respect patient autonomy, and ensure fair access to AI technologies.

Issues of Bias, Fairness, and Transparency

Biases can enter AI systems through data and algorithm design, the importance of fairness in AI applications, and the necessity for transparent methodologies. Recognizing and addressing these issues is critical for the ethical deployment of AI in healthcare.

AI Inherits and Amplifies Human Biases

Then, the chapter detailed the processes through which AI inherits biases and therefore AI applications trained on biased datasets can amplify these biases, leading to adverse outcomes. Understanding these mechanisms is crucial for clinicians to mitigate and prevent biased AI applications.

Overcoming Limitations of Ethical Use of AI

There are practical strategies to reduce biases, including diverse data collection, fairness-aware algorithms, and robust ethical frameworks. We also emphasized the importance of multidisciplinary collaboration in addressing these challenges effectively.

Call to Action

Clinicians, play a pivotal role in shaping the future of AI in healthcare. Advocacy for ethical AI and clinician active participation in its development, and vigilance in monitoring AI applications are crucial for ensuring that AI technologies serve all patients fairly and effectively. By championing diverse data inclusion, transparent methodologies, and continuous education on ethical AI practices, clinicians can help mitigate biases and promote equitable healthcare outcomes.

By embracing these responsibilities, clinicians will:

- Ensure Ethical AI Implementation: Advocate for and implement AI systems that adhere to ethical principles, reducing biases and promoting fairness.
- Foster Trust and Accountability: Build trust in AI technologies by ensuring transparency and accountability in their use.
- Drive Equitable Healthcare: Contribute to developing AI systems that provide equitable care for all patient populations, address historical disparities, and improve overall health outcomes.

Commitment to these goals will be instrumental in harnessing AI's full potential in healthcare, ensuring that it benefits all patients and upholds the highest ethical standards. Together, we can shape a future where AI in healthcare is both innovative and just.

Conclusion

In the rapidly evolving landscape of digital health, the integration of AI offers transformative potential, yet it also presents significant ethical challenges. This chapter explored the essential ethical principles of AI in healthcare, highlighted issues of bias, fairness, and transparency, examined how AI can inherit and amplify human biases, and reviewed case studies that illustrate these challenges. Finally, practical strategies for overcoming these limitations and ensuring the ethical use of AI were discussed.

References

1. Datatron. Real-life examples of discriminating artificial intelligence. Datatron. Published February 25, 2021. https://datatron.com/real-life-examples-of-discriminating-artificial-intelligence/#:~:text=COMPAS,defendant%20would%20become%20a%20recidivist. Accessed 29 June 2024.
2. Scientific American. Racial bias found in a major health care risk algorithm. Scientific American. Published October 24, 2019. https://www.scientificamerican.com/article/racial-bias-found-in-a-major-health-care-risk-algorithm/. Accessed 19 June 2024.
3. Jansen LA. Medical beneficence, nonmaleficence, and patients' well-being. J Clin Ethics. 2022;33(1):23–8.
4. Horowitz BT. How AI bias is impacting healthcare. InformationWeek. Published March 27, 2024. https://www.informationweek.com/machine-learning-ai/how-ai-bias-is-impacting-healthcare. Accessed 15 July 2024.
5. National Institutes of Health Revitalization Act of 1993. Public Law No: 103-43, 107 Stat. 122. June 10, 1993.
6. Epker E. June 10, 1993: 10 Facts about the NIH revitalization act as it turns 30. Forbes. Published June 6, 2023. https://www.forbes.com/sites/evaepker/2023/06/06/june-10-1993-10-facts-about-the-nih-revitalization-act-as-it-turns-30/. Accessed 15 July 2024.
7. Harvard Medical School Postgraduate Education. Embracing diversity: The imperative for inclusive clinical trials. Harvard Medical School Postgraduate Education. Published June 30, 2023. https://postgraduateeducation.hms.harvard.edu/trends-medicine/embracing-diversity-imperative-inclusive-clinical-trials. Accessed 29 June 2024.
8. U.S. Census Bureau. Quick Facts United States. https://census.gov/quickfacts/. Accessed 29 June 2024.
9. Steinberg JR, Turner BE, Weeks BT, Magnani CJ, Wong BO, Rodriguez F, et al. Analysis of female enrollment and participant sex by burden of disease in US clinical trials between 2000 and 2020. JAMA Netw Open. 2021;4(6):e2113749.
10. EurekAlert. Women underrepresented in clinical trials for key disease areas. EurekAlert. Published June 21, 2022. https://www.eurekalert.org/news-releases/956428. Accessed 29 June 2024.
11. Forbes Tech Council. Why diversity in health research is good science and good business. Forbes. Published February 28, 2022. https://www.forbes.com/sites/forbestechcouncil/2022/02/28/why-diversity-in-health-research-is-good-science-and-good-business/?sh=2feedf6d5cde. Accessed 15 July 2024.
12. Harvard Business Review. Eliminating algorithmic bias is just the beginning of equitable AI. Harvard Business Review. Published September 2023. https://hbr.org/2023/09/eliminating-algorithmic-bias-is-just-the-beginning-of-equitable-ai. Accessed 15 July 2024.
13. Vyas DA, Eisenstein LG, Jones DS. Hidden in plain sight—reconsidering the use of race correction in clinical algorithms. N Engl J Med. 2020;383(9):874–82.
14. PBS NewsHour. Understanding AI Bias in healthcare [Video]. YouTube. Published December 17, 2022. https://youtu.be/1O7Ov1nxMc0?si=yGmbh87v8vKHFHeh. Accessed 15 July 2024.
15. National Academies of Sciences, Engineering, and Medicine; Health and Medicine Division; Board on Population Health and Public Health Practice; Roundtable on the Promotion of Health Equity; Martinez RM, Taffe R, Alper J, eds. Examining the history, consequences, and effects of race-based clinical algorithms on health equity: proceedings of a workshop. Washington, DC: National Academies Press (US); December 27, 2023. https://www.ncbi.nlm.nih.gov/books/NBK600053/. Accessed 15 July 2024.
16. Anderson MA, Malhotra A, Non AL. Could routine race-adjustment of spirometers exacerbate racial disparities in COVID-19 recovery? Lancet Respir Med. 2021;9(2):124–5. Epub 2020 Dec 10.

17. Holder AL, Wong AI. The big consequences of small discrepancies: why racial differences in pulse oximetry errors matter. Crit Care Med. 2022;50(2):335–7.
18. Gichoya JW, Banerjee I, Bhimireddy AR, Burns JL, Celi LA, Chen LC, et al. AI recognition of patient race in medical imaging: a modelling study. Lancet Digit Health. 2022;4(6):e406–14. Epub 2022 May 11.
19. Pyrros A, Rodríguez-Fernández JM, Borstelmann SM, Gichoya JW, Horowitz JM, Fornelli B, et al. Detecting racial/ethnic health disparities using deep learning from frontal chest radiography. J Am Coll Radiol. 2022;19(1 Pt B):184–91.
20. PLOS Digital Health. Bias in artificial intelligence algorithms and recommendations for mitigation. PLOS Digital Health. Published June 22, 2023. https://journals.plos.org/digitalhealth/article?id=10.1371/journal.pdig.0000278. Accessed 15 July 2024.
21. Lolic M, Araojo R, Okeke M, Temple R. U.S. racial and ethnic participation in global clinical trials by therapeutic areas. J Clin Pharm Ther. 2021;46(6):1576–81.
22. STAT News. UnitedHealth pushed employees to follow an algorithm to cut off Medicare patients' rehab care. STAT News. Published November 14, 2023. https://www.statnews.com/2023/11/14/unitedhealth-algorithm-medicare-advantage-investigation/. Accessed 15 July 2024.
23. Healthcare Finance News. UnitedHealth AI algorithm allegedly led to Medicare Advantage denials, lawsuit claims. Healthcare Finance News. Published [Month Day, Year]. https://www.healthcarefinancenews.com/news/unitedhealth-ai-algorithm-allegedly-led-medicare-advantage-denials-lawsuit-claims. Accessed 15 July 2024.
24. Adedinsewo DA, Pollak AW, Phillips SD, Smith TL, Svatikova A, Hayes SN, et al. Cardiovascular disease screening in women: leveraging artificial intelligence and digital tools. Circ Res. 2022;130(4):673–90. Epub 2022 Feb 17.
25. The Guardian. Invisible women by Caroline Criado Perez—a world designed for men. The Guardian. Published February 28, 2019. https://www.theguardian.com/books/2019/feb/28/invisible-women-by-caroline-criado-perez-review. Accessed 15 July 2024.
26. Abramoff MD, Tarver ME, Loyo-Berrios N, Trujillo S, Char D, Obermeyer Z, Foundational Principles of Ophthalmic Imaging and Algorithmic Interpretation Working Group of the Collaborative Community for Ophthalmic Imaging Foundation, Washington, D.C.; Maisel WH, et al. Considerations for addressing bias in artificial intelligence for health equity. NPJ Digit Med. 2023;6(1):170. Published September 12, 2023.
27. American Medical Association. Principles for augmented intelligence development, deployment, and use. American Medical Association. https://www.ama-assn.org/system/files/ama-ai-principles.pdf. Accessed 15 July 2024.
28. World Health Organization. WHO releases AI ethics and governance guidance for large multi-modal models. World Health Organization. Published January 18, 2024. https://www.who.int/news/item/18-01-2024-who-releases-ai-ethics-and-governance-guidance-for-large-multi-modal-models. Accessed 15 July 2024.
29. Adams L, Fontaine E, Lin S, et al, editors. Artificial intelligence in health, health care, and biomedical science: an AI code of conduct framework principles and commitments discussion draft. NAM Perspectives. Commentary, National Academy of Medicine, Washington, DC; 2024.
30. GDPR.eu. What is GDPR, the EU's new data protection law? GDPR.eu. Published November 17, 2018. https://gdpr.eu/what-is-gdpr/. Accessed 19 June 2024.
31. Forbes. How to navigate the privacy crossroads between AI And HIPAA. Forbes. Published December 22, 2023. https://www.forbes.com/sites/shashankagarwal/2023/12/22/ai-and-hipaa-navigating-the-privacy-crossroads/. Accessed 15 July 2024.

Chapter 11
Artificial Intelligence Technology in Healthcare and the Digital Divide

Ranit Mishori

Introduction

The incorporation of Artificial Intelligence (AI)technologies into healthcare and clinical practice is promising on multiple levels, pushing the field—and ideally, outcomes—forward, with improved diagnostics, predictive analysis, personalized treatments, personalized education, and streamlining efficiencies in administrative tasks, among many other applications.

As we celebrate the promise, and caution about the excitement surrounding AI, we must also recognize the challenges and limitations, in the US and globally, specifically regarding access to these technologies and the risk of worsening existing inequities.

One area which deserves more attention is digital inclusion, or rather exclusion, in the context of what is known as the 'Digital Divide.' While AI-proponents tout the possibility of AI helping close disparities and bridging socio-economic gaps, others are more cautious, worrying that Digital Exclusion, or the Digital Divide, may be exacerbated with the emerging use of health-based generative-AI technologies and digital tools.

Scientists are raising concerns that AI technologies may be a "vehicle for the 'colonization of healthcare,' whereby the outputs enrich 'a powerful few by dispossessing communities that have been dispossessed before'" [1, 2]. Others note that "although generative AI technologies may be novel, early differences in uptake appear to be following familiar paths of digital marginalization" [3].

R. Mishori (✉)
Georgetown University School of Medicine, Washington, DC, USA
e-mail: mishorir@georgetown.edu

T. Adirim (ed.), *Digital Health, AI and Generative AI in Healthcare*,
https://doi.org/10.1007/978-3-031-83526-1_11

What Is the Digital Divide?

According to the Organization for Economic Co-operation and Development (OECD), the Digital Divide is the gap between individuals, households, businesses, and geographic areas at different socio-economic levels regarding both their opportunities to access Information and Communication Technologies (ICT) and to their use of the internet for a wide variety of activities [4].

Narrowing the focus to health, the World Health Organization notes that the digital divide in healthcare refers to the disparities in access to digital health technologies, which can lead to unequal health outcomes [5, 6].

Digitally excluded individuals or communities—with limited access to the internet, digital devices, or the skills to use these technologies—are at a disadvantage in receiving timely and effective healthcare services, exacerbating existing health inequalities. One recent example involves the early days of the rollout of the COVID-19 vaccine, whereas individuals with low tech literacy and no or limited connection to the internet were prevented from accessing vaccine appointments, despite being in an eligible priority group, such as those over the age of 65 [7].

Who Is Most at Risk for Experiencing a Digital Divide?

Certain individuals and communities are at risk for digital exclusion, due to elements closely associated with the Social Determinants of Health (SDOH) and factors related to socioeconomic status, age, gender, educational level, geographical setting, among others [8–10].

Historically, the digital divide has been associated with having limited financial resources. Limited or low-income status was shown to affect individuals' ability to access the internet, digital devices, and digital literacy resources. Communities and individuals living in rural areas are also affected and are often excluded from Information and Communication Technology (ICT) due to challenges with broadband infrastructure and cell tower distribution.

Age plays an important role, with older adults facing technical and digital literacy barriers, which may prevent them from engaging with digital and AI interfaces and programs. Computer and smartphone usage is lowest in the >65 years old age group [8–10].

Educational attainment is also linked to ICT use. Level of education is the strongest positive predictor of rates of search for generative AI tools. For example, research has shown that, in the US, counties with the highest rates of search for ChatGPT are more urbanized, educated and have more technology and creative sector jobs compared with the US overall [3].

People with disabilities (physical, sensory, cognitive) comprise another high-risk group, due to accessibility features that may be lacking in various digital and AI technologies [11].

Racial and ethnic minorities groups may be excluded from the benefits health-related digital innovation, such as AI, due to cultural and linguistic factors, as well as due to historical and contemporary marginalization and systemic discrimination.

Women, particularly in low-income countries, experience digital exclusion due to factors generally associated with pervasive gender discrimination which limits their access to digital tools and devices, results in lower tech literacy, and restricts their use of digital technology, including in healthcare [12].

Individuals and communities at the *intersection* of these factors, are even at greater risk of being excluded from digital life and all the benefits it may offer in education, commerce, employment, and health, among other areas.

Globally, the digital divide is clear when considering different geographical regions of the world where access to electricity and cell coverage, broadband infrastructure and overall technical adoption and digital penetration are far inferior in low-income compared to higher-income countries and the "Global North." Low-income, and developing countries, especially some in the African continent, parts of Southeast Asia and Latin America, have struggled to catch up and keep up with digital technology, including AI, due to low connectivity, prohibitive costs, and poor infrastructure. These disparities exacerbate and may deepen global inequalities in benefiting from health-sector advancements in digital and AI-based tools, as well as overall economic development [13].

Developing economies with struggling healthcare systems and insufficient digital infrastructure and limited capacity for innovation may not realize the same benefits and convenience from AI innovation as developed countries and more advanced healthcare systems.

Types, Causes and Drivers of the Digital Divide

Researchers have looked at digital exclusion, in general, via different frameworks, all focusing on the interconnectedness of various socio-economic factors. The factors associated with the digital divide can be viewed on or experienced at the individual level (e.g., a patient with certain characteristics), community level (e.g., certain marginalized groups), health-system level (e.g., private, academic, public), regional level (e.g., rural vs. urban), and global level (e.g., high-income vs. low-income country).

Wei et al. (2001) identified 3 levels of the Digital Divide: the first level, which identifies *access* to information technologies (e.g., in homes and schools), the second level, which focuses on *reduced capability* to use IT, arising from the first level, and other contextual factors; the third level focusing on a divide in *outcomes,* which arises from the lack of capability and poor access [14, 15].

Garcia-Martin and Garcia-Sanchez (2022), provide a variation of this framing, also identifying three factors responsible for the digital divide: (1) The lack of access to digital tools and internet connectivity; (2) The lack of digital literacy and instructional competencies; (3) The social and cultural disadvantages of not being involved on the world wide web [16].

Hilbert looks at the digital divide from the perspective of the individual experiencing digital exclusion and identifies four focal points: (1) the subject who accesses (who), (2) the subject's demographic characteristics, (3) the mode of connection (how), (4) the system the subject connects to. All are interrelated, he notes, and an unfavorable status in either one (or more) can lead to digital exclusion of certain individuals or communities [17].

Carter et al., add a 5th dimension that can contribute to engagement with ICT, particularly in the era of AI—the subject's perceptions and beliefs about the technology they are expected to engage with [15]. This relates to individual risk perception related to privacy and confidentiality in the health sector and may be informed by known biases involving certain groups of individuals (see Chap. 12).

Access

Access relates to the ability of certain individuals or populations to access the internet and/or other digital tools. Public facing advanced AI applications may require expensive hardware, and a reliable internet connection (via broadband, or cellular networks) is almost always a pre-requisite for use. Those may be unavailable to low-income communities, rural communities, or those with physical disabilities, thus preventing them from effective use of health-based AI tools.

For example, more than a third of the global population (greater than 2.9 billion people), do not have access to the internet [18, 19]. Such poor or non-existent access makes using AI technologies and healthcare solutions challenging if not impossible.

Another example is access to the hardware needed to access ICT or AI tools, such as computers or smart phones. According to data as of June 2024, while in the US more than 96% of the population owns smartphones, when you break it down by age group, only 46% of people over 65 do. Globally, a little less than 70% of the population owns a smartphone. Smartphone penetration by country, however, shows even greater gaps, where in some countries (e.g., Nigeria at 38%, Pakistan at 31%) most people don't own a smartphone [20, 21].

Living with a disability is another factor that influences accessibility. For example, individuals who are visually impaired, those with paraplegia, those affected by certain neurological disorders or amputees, might face challenges using or accessing digital technology or commonly available AI tools that require touch, vision, hearing, or that use facial features for use or identification [11].

Individuals or groups experiencing financial burdens may be unable to access to digital or AI technologies and tools, from having to pay monthly fees for internet providers, to cost prohibitive hardware (including the initial purchase to troubleshooting or maintenance costs). The cost of software licenses (initial or renewals), for individuals, institutions, or healthcare organizations (especially in low-income countries), will also determine their ability to engage with technological advances.

Beyond an individual's access issues related to their specific socio-economic factors, access is, importantly, influenced by policy factors, as well as regional or national infrastructure.

Many countries, particularly in the African continent, have daily challenges with electricity, unreliable energy sources, rolling blackouts, and load shedding, affecting individuals, schools, and healthcare facilities' ability to benefit from ICT and AI tools [22]. Cell phone coverage in many parts of the world can also be problematic, limiting individuals' ability to use smartphones equipped with AI tools [23].

Use (Literacy, Competency, or Capability)

Even if one has access to the right hardware, software, the internet and an area with good cell phone coverage, the ability to use specific health-related digital and AI technologies is related to digital and technical literacy, which is associated with the availability of education and training.

As is the case for general digital exclusion, low or a lack of digital literacy will prevent certain populations from benefitting from public or consumer facing health-AI technologies. This may particularly impact older adults, and communities experiencing low income and low general-literacy, English-literacy, or health-literacy.

This can be particularly important not only in relation to challenges with the technical use of advanced AI-tools, but also in response to AI-generated health mis- and dis-information, for example with the emergence of deepfakes, healthcare billing scams, and misleading/inaccurate treatment scams.

Teaching how to be discerning about the use of AI tools and content generated by generative-AI is critical. On the flip side, in cases where we would want people to use advantageous and "good" AI tools, individuals with general low-tech skills may have higher rates of suspicion about the technology, avoiding its use altogether [24, 25]. Training and education do exist, but marginalized communities may lack access to educational resources or face other constraints accessing training opportunities (e.g., transportation, money, time, English literacy in the context of the US).

Trust

Marginalized communities have historically been known to have lower levels of trust in the system, particularly the healthcare system. A combination of general distrust, with knowledge of the biases currently associated with various AI-tools, may result in a reluctance to adopt AI solutions, and a lower likelihood of certain individuals and groups engaging with newer health-AI tools, and benefitting from these potential advances [24, 25].

Data Inclusion and Exclusion

As described in Chaps. 5 and 10, AI systems often rely on training data that may exclude certain populations, thus introducing biases in the resulting guidance, recommendations, or interventions. This may also apply to health-based AI tools, where, historically, research comprises data based on decades of studies that excluded women, minorities, and individuals with disabilities, or that were carried out in English-speaking settings, excluding data from other parts of the world. Health-AI tools may also not factor differing practices and values related to health care interventions based on cultural or linguistic differences, potentially contributing to recommendations that may not be appropriate to certain groups.

From the user perspective, many AI tools are being developed in the English-language domain, affecting access of non-English speaking individuals from engaging with the new technology.

The Digital Determinants of Health

Researchers and policymakers have recognized the importance of raising awareness of the Digital Divide, the drivers that lead to it, and, ultimately, of the role of what is being termed the Digital Determinants of Health (DDOH) on the health outcomes of individuals and populations and on health equity in general [1, 26, 27].

Disparities in the adoption of Health AI tools and in overall digital access and skills as described above, can exacerbate existing health inequalities, particularly in marginalized populations. To achieve equitable health outcomes, we must address the Digital Determinants of Health [1, 26, 27].

Consideration of the DDOH should be expected and explicitly discussed throughout the design and roll out phases of artificial intelligence systems, and other forms of digital technology.

The digital exclusion risks are not new, and through adoption of mitigation measures at the individual, community, national and global levels we may be able to minimize the impact of the digital divide and of digital exclusion related to health-AI tools and applications.

Digital Divide Risk Mitigation/Digital Inclusion

Digital inclusion interventions in health-AI exist on a continuum of stakeholders that includes the patient, the health professional or clinician, the health system, the research, and development sector, in the context of national and regional geopolitics.

Interventions could include implementation of policies by governments to ensure access to broadband, cellular coverage, the internet, devices and health-based AI technologies; On the research and development side, designers and developers should be encouraged and incentivized to focus on inclusive design that considers population diversity, from the physical, linguistic, and cultural perspective.

Digital inclusion must also consider *who* is involved in developing new AI tools. The inclusion of women and technologists/developers/scientists from the Global South, would likely enhance content development, cultural humility, bias reduction, and trust in the emerging tools and products.

Community engagement should be key throughout the development process of AI technologies,, hardware, tools, and interfaces. At-risk communities should be consulted early in the development process about their needs and preferences. Such efforts could also help build trust which may result in enhanced adoption and acceptance of consumer and patient-facing AI tools and systems.

Enhancing digital literacy, especially of at-risk populations, must be part of any efforts to expand acceptability and engagement with AI technologies and tools. Education and training programs may help build digital skills and enable exposure of more individuals and communities to AI-based health technologies, ultimately allowing them to benefit from these innovations.

The Role of Health Professionals

As healthcare professionals we have a responsibility to be aware of the Digital Determinants of Health, understand how they intersect with the SDOH, and appreciate how these drivers may exclude patients and communities from benefiting from the expanding array of innovative AI solutions in healthcare. We also have a role in educating patients about digital literacy and helping them navigate AI tools.

We must understand and be able to explain the limitations of AI tools related to the training data they are based on and resist the hype.

We must work with developers to ensure AI training data reflects the diversity of our patient populations, both domestically and globally. We can be advocates for ethical use, human rights and safety standards, privacy safeguards, and help shape policies and regulations of AI tools and technologies that seek to minimize the digital divide.

Health system researchers, with the collaboration of Health-AI Tech developers and companies, must develop and implement a research agenda that evaluates the use and impact of AI tools on communities at risk for digital exclusion.

The World Benchmarking Alliance has developed helpful benchmarks for digital inclusion for companies and developers, some of which may be adopted to the healthcare system. Those benchmarks can be found at: https://www.worldbenchmarkingalliance.org/digital-inclusion-benchmark/ [28].

By taking these actions, health professionals can promote the development and use of AI technologies and tools that enhance equity and inclusion, reduce the risk of deepening or exacerbating the digital divide, and ultimately, improve health outcomes for all.

Conclusion

Promoting 'AI for Good' means recognizing how digital exclusion affects individuals and populations, and safeguarding against situations in which the benefits of AI in healthcare could inequitably favor those who are already advantaged and privileged, widening health gaps, and deepening inequities associated with the social drivers of health.

Health professionals can be leaders in creating the right conditions where "no one is left behind," reflecting the UN Sustainable Development Goals commitment to ensure that all people, especially the most marginalized, benefit from global progress.

References

1. Chidambaram S, Jain B, Jain U, Mwavu R, Baru R, Thomas B, et al. An introduction to digital determinants of health. PLOS Digit Health. 2024;3(1):e0000346.
2. Artificial intelligence is creating a new colonial world order. MIT Technology Review. https://www.technologyreview.com/2022/04/19/1049592/artificial-intelligence-colonialism/. Accessed 10 Aug 2024.
3. Daepp MIG, Counts S. The emerging AI divide in the United States. Published online April 30, 2024.
4. OECD, Understanding the digital divide, OECD Digital Economy Papers, No. 49, 2001. Paris: OECD Publishing.
5. AI risks in global health 'must be accounted for'—WHO. https://www.gavi.org/vaccineswork/ai-risks-global-health-must-be-accounted-who. Accessed 10 Aug 2024.
6. World Health Organization. Global strategy on digital health 2020–2025. Geneva: World Health Organization; 2021.
7. Mishori, R. To vaccinate America, close the digital divide. https://thehill.com/opinion/healthcare/536085-to-vaccinate-america-close-the-digital-divide/. Accessed 10 Aug 2024.
8. Mishori R, Antono B. Telehealth, rural America, and the digital divide. J Ambul Care Manage. 2020;43(4):319–22.
9. Reddy H, Joshi S, Joshi A, Wagh V. A critical review of global digital divide and the role of technology in healthcare. Cureus. 14(9):e29739.
10. Makri A. Bridging the digital divide in health care. Lancet Digit Health. 2019;1(5):e204–5.
11. Welker Y. Council post: algorithmic diversity: mitigating AI bias and disability exclusion. Forbes. https://www.forbes.com/sites/forbestechcouncil/2023/05/09/algorithmic-diversity-mitigating-ai-bias-and-disability-exclusion/. Accessed 11 Aug 2024.
12. I'd blush if I could: closing gender divides in digital skills through education—UNESCO Digital Library. https://unesdoc.unesco.org/ark:/48223/pf0000367416. Accessed 11 Aug 2024.
13. The World Bank. Digital progress and trends report. https://www.worldbank.org/en/publication/digital-progress-and-trends-report. Accessed 11 Aug 2024.
14. Wei KK, Teo HH, Chan HC, Tan BCY. Conceptualizing and testing a social cognitive model of the digital divide. Inf Syst Res. 2011;22(1):170–87.
15. Carter L, Liu D, Cantrell C. Exploring the intersection of the digital divide and artificial intelligence: a hermeneutic literature review. AIS Trans Human-Comput Interact. 2020;12(4):253–75.
16. García-Martín J, García-Sánchez JN. The digital divide of know-how and use of digital technologies in higher education: the case of a college in Latin America in the COVID-19 Era. Int J Environ Res Public Health. 2022;19(6):3358.

17. Hilbert M. Digital divide(s). In: The international Encyclopedia of digital communication and society. Hoboken: Wiley; 2015. p. 1–7. https://doi.org/10.1002/9781118767771.wbiedcs012.
18. UN Agency for digital technologies. Facts and Figures 2021: 2.9 billion people still offline. ITU. November 29, 2021. https://www.itu.int/hub/2021/11/facts-and-figures-2021-2-9-billion-people-still-offline/. Accessed 11 Aug 2024.
19. Mishori, R, Hampton K. Broadband is a human right—the medical care blog. https://www.themedicalcareblog.com/broadband-is-a-human-right/. Accessed 10 Aug 2024.
20. Global smartphone penetration 2016–2023. Statista. https://www.statista.com/statistics/203734/global-smartphone-penetration-per-capita-since-2005/. Accessed 11 Aug 2024.
21. How many people own smartphones? (2024–2029). Exploding topics. November 19, 2021. https://explodingtopics.com/blog/smartphone-stats. Accessed 11 Aug 2024.
22. World Bank Open Data. World Bank Open Data. https://data.worldbank.org. Accessed 11 Aug 2024.
23. UN Agency for Digital Technologies. Facts and Figures 2023—mobile network coverage. https://www.itu.int/itu-d/reports/statistics/2023/10/10/ff23-mobile-network-coverage. Accessed 11 Aug 2024.
24. Bentley SV, Naughtin CK, McGrath MJ, Irons JL, Cooper PS. The digital divide in action: how experiences of digital technology shape future relationships with artificial intelligence. AI Ethics. Published online March 18, 2024.
25. Naughtin C, Bentley SV. The 'digital divide' is already hurting people's quality of life. Will AI make it better or worse? The Conversation. March 19, 2024. http://theconversation.com/the-digital-divide-is-already-hurting-peoples-quality-of-life-will-ai-make-it-better-or-worse-222987. Accessed 10 Aug 2024.
26. Governing Health Futures 2030. The digital determinants of health: policy brief. https://governinghealthfutures2030.org/pdf/policy-briefs/DigitalDeterminants.pdf. Accessed 11 Aug 2024.
27. Holmes Fee C, Hicklen RS, Jean S, Abu Hussein N, Moukheiber L, de Lota MF, et al. Strategies and solutions to address digital determinants of health (DDOH) across underinvested communities. PLOS Digit Health. 2023;2(10):e0000314.
28. World Benchmarking Alliance. 2023 Digital Inclusion Benchmark Insights Report. Published March 2023. https://www.worldbenchmarkingalliance.org/research/2023-digital-inclusion-benchmark-insights-report/. Accessed 14 Aug 2024.

Chapter 12
Privacy and Legal Issues in the Use of Artificial Intelligence

Karen Habercoss

Introduction

The volume of health information globally produced, acquired, and copied is projected to continue increasing from approximately 64.2 zettabytes in 2020 to the addition of possibly another 180 zettabytes by 2025 [1]. For context, one zettabyte is enormous, it's the equivalent of one trillion gigabytes. Health data consumed for artificial intelligence (AI) primarily uses information generated from past and current patients, individual consumers who have yet to become or may never be a future patient of an entity, and in some cases biomedical research of human subjects. Each of these data types and the purposes for use and processing can be regulated and controlled by distinct legal requirements, governmental directives, externally developed professional frameworks, methodologies or guidelines, and internal entity-specific governance.

AI generally requires large amounts of quality data to assure the integrity of outputs [2]. AI is a technology that requires a clinician's privacy support just like all other types of health information technology. The larger the data cohort the more chance for a privacy incident caused by mismanagement, unintentional misuse, or in the extreme, maliciousness, especially without good oversight. Patients and the public are becoming ever more attentive to the sensitive nature of health data. They want their health information used in compliance with the law, with greater transparency and control, and they expect being informed of how their data are shared with others, even when used among health professionals, and the technologies used to share it [3].

Healthcare organizations are expected to analyze and understand the risks of their data acquisition, use, and sharing. This often means garnering patient approval as required or whenever possible and acting in accordance with applicable

K. Habercoss (✉)
The University of Chicago Medicine, Chicago, IL, USA

T. Adirim (ed.), *Digital Health, AI and Generative AI in Healthcare*,
https://doi.org/10.1007/978-3-031-83526-1_12

information privacy rights in ways that providers may not have previously considered. Organizational and professional eagerness for innovation must be balanced with careful consideration of individual privacy rights. According to a Pew Research Center study, "Though Americans can identify a mix of pros and cons regarding the use of AI in health and medicine, caution remains a dominant theme in public views. When it comes to the pace of technological adoption, three-quarters of Americans say their greater concern is that health care providers will move too fast implementing AI in health and medicine before fully understanding the risks for patients; far fewer (23%) say they are more concerned that providers will move too slowly, missing opportunities to improve patients' health" [4].

Recognition that AI is meant to support, not substitute, a clinician's medical decision-making is an important concept [5]. This idea, along with continuous evaluation by the clinician of AI use cases involving health data for purpose and privacy impact, are one blueprint that can be used to enhance patient and consumer trust. Trust is to be regarded through both the lens of the AI technological capabilities themselves and within the clinician, research, or entity itself using AI to support care of the patient [6]. Clinical providers and leaders of healthcare entities augment confidence when they have a baseline understanding of the important techniques used by privacy professionals to protect confidentiality. These supports can include data mapping to understand the internal and external flows of data, privacy, and security by design to protect and secure data in systems, and the use of privacy enhancing technologies to further safeguard individually identifiable data and promote integrity.

Legal and Regulatory Frameworks Governing AI in Healthcare

The use of new technologies in healthcare, including AI, has been accompanied by an increasing awareness of data privacy considerations. In the U.S., AI has not yet been subjected to fully updated analyses and interpretations of existing laws for applicability. Only recently have federal and state governments considered whether new regulations are needed to provide guardrails on its use. Clinicians will need to be mindful that the AI regulatory and legal landscape is in its infancy. Commonly, data acquisitions, uses, processing, and disclosures fall into categories of required, permissible with and/or without the need for consent or authorization, and impermissible. Considerations for possibly applicable privacy and data protection regulations, directives, and principles are shown in Table 12.1. Whether these apply could be dependent upon the AI purpose and source of the data within healthcare. Health professionals of all types are strongly encouraged to work directly with their designated privacy officials or counsel to assess all legal and regulatory obligations at the federal, state, and international levels. It is vital to know how one may be subject to relevant, new AI laws, recently created statutes and directives, as well as all other

Table 12.1 Healthcare data used for artificial intelligence: privacy and data protection regulations, directives, and principal considerations

Name	Country
United States Health Insurance Portability and Accountability Act (HIPAA)	United States
Executive Order on the Safe, Secure, and Trustworthy Development and Use of Artificial Intelligence	United States
Blueprint for an AI Bill of Rights	United States
Health Information Technology for Economic and Clinical Health Act (HITECH)	United States
21st Century Cures Act	United States
Confidentiality of Substance Use Disorder Patient Records (42 CFR Part 2)	United States
Family Educational Rights and Privacy Act (FERPA)	United States
Genetic Information Nondiscrimination Act (GINA)	United States
General Data Protection Regulation (GDPR)	European Union and United Kingdom
Artificial Intelligence Act	European Union
Digital Services Act	European Union
Personal Information Protection Law (PIPL)	China
Personal Information Protection and Electronic Documents Act (PIPEDA)	Canada
The Privacy Act	Canada
Digital Personal Data Protection Act (DPDP)	India
The General Data Protection Law (LGPD)	Brazil
Social Principles of Human-Centric AI	Japan
Civil Rights Act of 1964	United States
Children's Online Privacy Protection Rule (COPPA)	United States
Other laws and regulatory considerations: Equal Employment Opportunity Commission (Automated Decision Making); Federal Trade Commission (Antitrust; Consumer Protection; Unfair or Deceptive Acts or Practices); Occupational Safety and Health Administration (Robotics); US individual state laws; Global laws	United States and Other Global

known healthcare business functional requirements to prevent any potential prospective regulatory or legal consequences of being found to not be compliant with obligations. Non-compliance may lead to monetary penalties, corrective actions with enhanced oversight, and/or public erosion of trust in a professional or personal brand.

The healthcare and public health sectors are highly regulated and designated as one of the U.S. government's sixteen critical infrastructure sectors [7]. The main privacy law governing a clinician's use of health data in the United States has historically been at the federal level through The Health Insurance Portability and Accountability Act (HIPAA) of 1996 [8]. It has had subsequent associated modifications, amendments, and updates to its privacy, security, and breach rules. It has also been strengthened through additional laws such as the Health Information

Technology for Economic and Clinical Health Act (HITECH) seeking to increase technological efficiency and the 21st Century Cures Act endorsing interoperability among other components, all in the interest of promoting patient safety and quality of care.

HIPAA requires those noted to be covered entities (most healthcare providers, health plans, and healthcare clearinghouses) and third party vendors performing certain types of services on behalf of these covered entities (business associates), to follow its privacy, security, and breach rules for uses and disclosures of individually identifiable health information, including its subset of patient protected health information, and de-identified information which is not attributable back to an individual person [9]. For those employed in healthcare, the use of identifiable patient information within a publicly available AI tool, for example, would require each patient to sign a valid written authorization to allow the individual health data as an input, otherwise it may implicate a violation of the law. HIPAA covered entities may be permitted to use a business associate agreement with a vendor when using an enterprise level AI technology to perform a covered service on their behalf, thus written patient permission may not be required. Use of fully de-identified or anonymized patient health data to support AI tools may be allowable without authorization or a business associate contractual agreement. However, clinicians must have strong knowledge of what constitutes de-identification or anonymization under the law to remain complaint. Rules and regulations at the U.S. federal level that should be considered for health data use within AI technology include those drafted and enforced by the: Department of Health and Human Services through the Office Civil Rights (OCR), Office of Inspector General (OIG), or Substance Abuse and Mental Health Services Administration (SAMHSA); Federal Trade Commission (FTC); Department of Education; Food and Drug Administration (FDA); Office of the National Coordinator (ONC); Centers for Medicare and Medicaid Services (CMS); Equal Employment Opportunity Commission (EEOC); Occupational Safety and Health Administration (OSHA); Office of the Attorney General (AG); US Department of Justice (DOJ); and others.

Healthcare institutions and businesses have become systems that span multiple states or even worldwide facilitating the rise of medical tourism, telehealth options, widespread promotional information, and education services, and increasing international research collaborations [10]. All of this makes the regulatory landscape for a healthcare provider or biological science researcher more complex than ever, especially with states like California and Washington having the California Consumer Privacy Act, the California Privacy Rights Act, and the Washington My Health My Data Act function as examples. The acquisition, processing, use, and disclosure of health data for AI is no longer viewable just in the context of HIPAA. It is now also encompassing a variety of other current and future federal, individual state and international laws, principles, and governmental directives. This requires each AI use case to be carefully understood in advance. Health professionals need to consider how they will use their own patient's trusted data within the context of an individual level in which they have a trusted treatment relationship with the person. Differentially, can the data be de-identified, anonymized, can aggregate health data be used instead, what, or how much will be used, and whether the data are patient, consumer, or research related.

State specific privacy laws currently, or soon to be enacted, can apply to individually identifiable health data in some cases where HIPAA may not. Most of the currently passed state privacy laws have implications for the access and use of data at the consumer level that could be triggered, for example, when collecting data through health-related websites, applications, or other education and marketing forms, particularly from individuals who are not patients [11]. In mid-2024, Colorado became the first state to pass a consumer law specific to AI. As of early 2024, about 25% of US states are considering the regulation of AI through a new law [12]. Other countries are also considering or have passed laws and principles for the use of AI. For example, the European Union's (EU) General Data Protection Regulation (GDPR), currently one of the world's strictest data privacy and security laws, already characterizes health data as sensitive and thus necessitates people be given certain legally noted and enforceable privacy rights for this as well as for research data [13]. Many new and currently developing AI regulations are risk based. Clinicians would do well to begin to consider, if not already, what current risks their own artificial intelligence usage poses.

With the recent passage of the EU AI Act, tiers have been developed to implement rules for assessing privacy risk in AI technologies as high, limited, and minimal, and with some even being considered completely unacceptable and disallowable [14]. There are more stringent rules for AI systems considered to be of higher risk. Clinicians must be aware of where health data are originating and the purpose prior to use in AI technologies, especially considering extraterritorial jurisdiction of some regulations. Those who operate in healthcare will also need to be mindful of AI relational to other countries' current and emerging requirements promoting responsible innovation aside from just the EU, including but not limited to Canada and its Artificial Intelligence and Data Act (AIDA), the Artificial Intelligence Law of the People's Republic of China, and privacy laws in Brazil and India to assure compliance. Healthcare professionals, including researchers, will encounter and use AI technologies given the increasing rates these are being implemented. The responsibility to protect privacy and act in compliance with regulations, directives, and principles is fundamental to the patient relationship, and requires clinicians to ask questions about how data of their own patients are being procured and used to train or even enhance models of purchased AI technologies.

In late 2023, a U.S. Presidential Executive Order was issued that initiated, among other things, the prospective for privacy standards for AI to build trust and manage risk through safe and secure appraisals of systems [15]. Clinicians must also consider highly confidential data types entered and used in AI as well as how bias and ethics may play a part in the outputs. Many AI systems use automation to increase efficiencies. The technological processes should remain consistent with data privacy principles.

The Nature of Sensitive Information in Healthcare

AI technologies in healthcare have the potential to learn, evolve, and support clinical decision making from private and sensitive data. Health information itself is sensitive by its very nature because it is individualized. However, there can be subjectivity related to the degree to which each person believes their own or others health information might be categorized as sensitive and the level of privacy that it should be afforded. Privacy is an essential principle in healthcare and almost every health professional organization, including the American Medical Association, recognizes upholding privacy as a precondition of maintaining trust in the clinical relationship [16]. People engage in health care or participate in research expecting to have the clinician or investigator keep the intimate details shared during the interactions or collected as part of the experience safe and confidential. Additionally, health information designated as especially sensitive requires extra care when handling by a clinician and may trigger additional legal obligations for the provider during its use or disclosure outside the treatment relationship. This type of information falls into categories the public may perceive as personally distressing or causing reputational damage if privacy is breached, most especially at the individual level. These can also be specifically defined and governed in and of themselves under state, federal, and international laws.

These categorical areas of sensitive health data necessitating supplementary forethought for use in AI technologies can include, but are not limited to: mental health and developmental disability, substance use, genetics and genomics, reproductive medicine, communicable diseases such as HIV and AIDS and other sexually transmitted diseases, gender and sexual identity, child or elder abuse and neglect, domestic violence, and sexual assault. Each has the potential for risky privacy concerns if not adequately accounted for in AI, especially when training models. There is great value placed on safeguarding an individual's privacy and how information is shared across a continuum of personal, social, professional, and financial manners, and many times health information is the most personal [17]. Release of sensitive health information can even lead to bias or discrimination and harm [18].

Assuring highly confidential types of information within electronic health records, insurance payment systems, research databases, and other data sets containing health information are tagged as restricted, and then segmented from other non-sensitive data sources, is a way for health providers and researchers to identify where these special kinds of data may exist. Sensitive data can be protected and disclosures of data for AI purposes can be better analyzed when appropriately identified. For example, patients with mental health conditions may have distinct privacy reservations than other patients do about sharing information [19]. Coding and isolating more sensitive types of data can offer additional privacy protections when used in conjunction with AI technologies. When developing and training AI models or using sensitive data within already developed technologies containing AI, there must be a level of trust and assurance proportional to this data type given the potential for individual discomfort that could arise if there was leakage of personal information, no matter how inadvertent. Patients and research subjects do not want their information misused or ineffectively accounted for thus causing them emotional harm or reputational damage.

Another source of sensitive health information to consider is patient searches on health care websites. The internet is increasingly used to explore health conditions and identify care providers. A study by White and Horvitz noted that one of eight web searches where there is intention to use healthcare will result in care being sought and, not surprisingly, the timing of this is based upon how serious the symptoms being searched are believed to be [20]. Sensitive health conditions could have a symptom acuity higher than others could. Delicate and complex personal topics may be searched via the internet and entered into forms or scheduling applications on a health clinician's professional website all while seeking or following through with services. The clinician should have advanced knowledge of any AI technology operating by potential third parties on their website, which could in turn use the patient entered information for continuous training of the third-party product. The patient may choose telehealth options that connect through the web to protect privacy. Internet connected sites should be evaluated with an elevated level of due diligence to ascertain whether AI is enabled and could pose potential privacy concerns. Healthcare institutions and clinical professionals should be cautious within their websites that may contain or interact with AI technologies especially if sensitive health information resides or is captured there to ensure this information is not passed through to unknown sources and that patient privacy protections remain in place. Considerations of patient confidentiality in AI used in consumer based, publicly available, informational, or educational websites, web-based patient portals, telehealth settings, and online payment environments are important but often forgotten by clinicians.

Consent and Data Sharing in the Context of AI Applications

Considerations for data acquisition, access, use, processing, and/or disclosure in AI should begin with the question - what is the purpose? It is often the answer to this initial contextual question that will inform the correct privacy requirements and whether a privacy professional should be engaged to complete an impact assessment. If that purpose changes, a re-evaluation should take place to assure the clinician understands the risks. Upfront, it is important when clinicians are starting to use a new AI tool or model to discern if the patient health information being used through inputs and outputs will be reused throughout multiple models or technologies or used for secondary purposes by either a vendor or researcher. Purposes can include clinical patient support including direct treatment, payment, or institutional-level operational health workflows involving quality improvement. They might also involve life sciences research or consumer experiences such as informal learning about treatment options or access to care information. According to Deloitte, 48%

of health consumers in a recent survey personally use generative AI themselves, with well-being being one of the main reasons [21].

As the purpose of any new AI use case is contemplated, the level and type of data needs to be understood. This means knowing whether individually identifiable data entered into the technology by the clinician will be used in any other manner, not originally expected, by the company that owns the AI technology. It also means determining if identifiable data will be completely de-identified or anonymized later for a secondary purpose or if data of many individuals will be combined to form an aggregate data set for use by some other party.

When an individual is recognizable, in most healthcare cases, a written authorization must be obtained from the individual prior to use of the data outside of the clinical care relationship between the clinician and patient. This written permission would need to follow the regulatory requirements for the use case and would need to describe the purpose in plain language. When possible, AI developers should be highly encouraged, by clinicians purchasing a product, to use de-identified or anonymized data in compliance with those same regulatory requirements, or if it is used in aggregate, clinicians must understand whether consent is required or should be attained as best practice. The granularity of the authorization or consent should always follow applicable laws. In situations where health providers and researchers are using vendors to perform services, sharing data into outside technologies, or are collaborating with external third parties, appropriate contractual arrangements should be put in place accurately denoting data use parameters and sharing obligations, and in many cases these agreements are required by law.

Large data sets for AI can pose specific challenges for practitioners and researchers in ascertaining what manner to incorporate informed consent [22]. The important aspect of informed consent deserving of attention is the patient, research subject, or health consumer must be provided advanced knowledge of which information is being used, at what level of detail, how it is used, by whom, and for how long, all in a way that is fully understandable. As part of consent, health data should only be collected, used, shared, and retained for as long as necessary and to fulfill the agreed upon purpose. This privacy concept of data minimization exists and is required in almost every jurisdiction. Within technology systems, the professional's inquiry is how to limit data to respect privacy while at the same time maximizing the design and data consumption to enhance functionality to offer the desired outcome of health benefit, and this involves going back to the query of purpose and understanding the data [23].

Risks to Patient Privacy and Privacy Incidents in Healthcare Settings

Patient, health consumer, and human subject research types of privacy risks for AI can have severe consequences if not proactively planned, managed, and monitored. Poorly managed risks can lead to data breaches with penalties imposed on the clinician or their organization and loss of trust by patients. Specifically, the use of unapproved, unsanctioned, or untested AI technologies in addition to the unauthorized use of distinguishable data can lead to information security incidents or exposures of individually identifiable health information and its subsets of protected health information or highly confidential information when data categories are not known, accounted for, or are misunderstood. This can apply to enterprise technologies, internally developed models and tools, and most predominantly in AI tools that are publicly available. Regardless of whether impermissible data repercussions are inadvertent or not, the significance of potential regulatory, legal, and financial implications remain. Data that are well governed offers clinicians' direction during all sequences of the AI lifecycle process as a way to appreciate risks [24]. Examples of governance can take the form of: policies and procedures that indicate acceptable uses of AI by clinicians, educating and providing guidance to healthcare providers about how to minimally assess and ask certain pertinent questions about the AI technologies they use within their organization, and having clinicians chair or be involved and part of AI oversight steering committees within a healthcare entity.

Classifying and categorizing, not only data types, but also privacy risks cannot be stagnant, and it is a process requiring maturity as AI technology usage evolves [25]. The ability to re-identify or geo-locate discrete people without expressed permission or through an approved transparent means, and the ability attribute their sensitive health information back to them individually, is one of the biggest risks clinicians face, as there would be no expectancy of direct details being publicly available. This type of internal or external data leakage can lead to unauthorized access, use, processing or disclosures, misuses of data, spillage of additional information, or unintended availability of data related to genetically related family members causing compliance issues for the provider. Depending on the types of impermissible information accessible, data leakage can lead to actual data breaches under one of the many previously mentioned federal, state, or international laws. Any identified data breach will have regulatory reporting requirements. Breaches of over 500 unique individuals under the U.S. federal HIPAA regulation or noncompliance with data subject rights under the EU GDPR will also trigger additional breach reporting obligations in healthcare. In breach cases, a loss of patient trust can move downstream to the direct clinician.

AI privacy risks that require clinician consideration are categorized as invasion risks, data collection risks, dissemination risks, and data processing risks [24]. Data collection risks can involve surveillance, observations of individuals without their knowledge or understanding [24]. Data dissemination risks can include the previously mentioned impermissible release of data, the alteration of health information leading to quality of care or financial issues, and the increased availability of health information to workforce members who may not have a need to know [24]. Data processing risks may involve the ability to relink health information to a patient, consumer, or research participant and may include data aggregation when this could allow individual corollaries [24]. It can also involve using data for a purpose beyond the original intent, also called secondary use, not providing advanced communication about the use case purpose, or even negligence in the extreme [24].

The overall risk of information security and cybersecurity events in healthcare is growing in frequency and nature. The health sector is under constant threat from not only global threats, including nation state threat actors, but unfortunately also by internal malicious workforce. The use of AI enhanced based attacks is of emerging concern because of the increasing ease of development and deployment against healthcare providers, payers, and third-party vendors with significant financial, reputational, and patient confidence damage as the result. An intrusion into the AI system resulting in a compromise of data is an example of an invasion risk [24]. All clinicians and their healthcare institutions must remain on high alert and take steps to proactively secure health information to prevent a downstream privacy incident.

Innovation Versus Individual Privacy Rights

Much of healthcare is based upon interpersonal reliance developed during human interactions. The notion of transparency of use by the clinician becomes an increasingly important privacy right when balancing the complexities of AI advancements. It is important for individuals to grasp when and how AI is being used, why it was chosen to fulfill certain efforts, what areas it is being planned, trained, and deployed, how it is examined and restructured over time, and eventually when it should no longer be needed [26]. Stored data accumulated from various sources such as electronic medical records and other health repositories, implantable devices, personal wearables and body sensors, mobile phones, genomic sequencing, and medical imaging can be aggregated, combined, and used to process, analyze, and make higher level predictions [27]. Clinicians and patients alike are often caught unready and unprepared for the extent of data acquisition sources and methods.

These particular uses of big data analytics could allow multiple patients to share their own personal health data with providers to further drive outcomes used by AI, as long as patients are told and understand that what they provide might be repurposed. Initially, an individual may share data with their primary clinician to assist with current medical care. As data are obtained and ingested into a patient health record, a secondary use may involve consolidating and aggregating larger sets of data for other innovations related to the treatment of many, generalizable research, greater public health efforts, or consumer driven insights. Respect for privacy of these secondary purposes is significant, as is the need to assure that the quality and integrity of the data remain intact. Patients, research subjects, and healthcare consumers commonly retain privacy rights under the law, and certainly at minimum as a best practice, related to the acquisition of, the access to, the use, processing and disclosure of, and the ability to request to amend health information as it relates to them individually regardless of the platform.

Specific categories and types of rights are often required by a federal, state, or international statute, but can even more generally be the standards used to inform these laws by the Fair Information Practice Principles (FIPPs) [28]. FIPPs are established privacy values that healthcare professionals can keep in mind and use to provide a critical sense of balance in AI advancement. These include: individual access to information about oneself and a manner to correct inaccuracies; accountability to applicable regulations and ways to observe compliance with these including adequate training of workforce; adherence to the authority to "create, collect, use, process, store, maintain, disseminate, or disclose" data; an advanced appreciation of a defined purpose and then using only the minimum necessary amount of data to perform just that actual task at hand in a way that is precise, suitable, pertinent, and complete; recognition of the method to obtain consent or authorization from the person when applicable or required and a grievance or inquiry procedure related to this if errors or concerns arise; setting up administrative, technical, and physical safeguards to maintain data security in advance; and offering notification detailing the transparency and availability of data privacy rights in plain language, no higher than a fifth grade reading level [28].

Navigating and Overcoming Challenges

Given the multitude of privacy regulatory and legal considerations with AI in healthcare, there are ways to oversee and control challenges. The first step is to allow a privacy professional to perform and share results of data mapping to understand where all types of health-related data are sourcing and originating from and how it flows through internal and external institutional systems and business processes. This can be presented back to the clinician in a visual format and should include notations of data maintenance, retention, and destruction in the movement throughout the lifecycle of the health information to inform. Governance through a well-developed framework can then be put into practice by the clinician's entity. The National Institute of Standards and Technology (NIST) has both privacy and AI frameworks that offer healthcare institutions and their clinicians a formal structure to manage and mitigate risks. The NIST privacy framework provides a way to initiate negotiation toward privacy outcomes, a method of operational prioritization, and a way to view associated risks in the larger business context [29]. The NIST AI framework, when used in conjunction with the privacy framework, can offer a means to responsibly plan, cultivate, organize, and put forth use cases for AI within a risk-based perspective [30]. Providers want to make certain the privacy professionals they work with explain the framework areas most beneficial to their individual clinical practice.

The widely accepted global concept of Privacy by Design was initiated by Ann Cavoukian at the Office of the Information and Privacy Commissioner of Ontario. It is one that emphasizes the importance of embedding comprehensive privacy specific principles into technologies and business plans from the start as a way to safeguard data. Privacy by Design involves exploring preventive measures, building privacy protective ideologies into the entire lifespan, showing respect for individual choice options, openly considering all user requirements, and complementing all appropriate interests as main selections [31]. Asking about the use of Privacy by

Design within AI models being developed or technologies purchased from third party vendors is another way to consider and adhere to known privacy doctrines and strengthen efforts.

Using privacy enhancing technologies, see Table 12.2, such as synthetic data for training AI data sets, may successfully and ably increase AI resilience in biological sciences research and clinical AI technology developments, and it can address confidentiality and security concerns. Synthetic data are similar to real data because they maintain the associations of data variables and is mathematically equivalent but fully preserves privacy by not having actual linkages to real individuals and is becoming an alternative for healthcare and research uses in AI, especially modeling; because it is not real individual data, there is greater ease of sharing which in turn opens additional AI prospects for usage [32]. Other electronic based tools called privacy enhancing technologies (PETs) can be used to protect information during acquisition, processing, and examination as a means to navigate regulations [33]. The PET can secure privacy either by cryptographic or statistical ways, both protecting data. Very generally, cryptography concentrates on encryption techniques, while statistics make changes in the data. In some cases, the PET, for example homomorphic encryption or differential privacy, alters the exemplification to offer safeguards by concealing sensitive details [34]. Homomorphic encryption is a coding method that can allow calculations without having to decrypt and expose real data. Differential privacy, used for large sensitive data, uses mathematical practices to bring in randomness to the data set while preserving the eventual outcome analysis. In other cases, the PET may change the calculation setting parameters as a precaution, such as with multiparty computation where data are shared with integrity but do not expose the underlying information [34]. Dependent upon the use cases and types of sensitive patient, human subjects research, or health consumer data desired for AI, PETs are gaining ground as a method to offer security and protections. They can also be used to share very large amounts of non-identifiable data from one industry to another to assist in healthcare research and training of open-source models that can be used to develop AI products used by health professionals in clinical practice.

Table 12.2 Types of privacy enhancing technologies

Privacy enhancing technology examples	Type
Differential Privacy	Cryptographic
Federated Learning	Statistical
Homomorphic Encryption	Cryptographic
Multiparty Computation	Cryptographic
Synthetic Data	Statistical
Zero-Knowledge Proofs	Cryptographic

Conclusion

AI has the capability to transform how medicine is currently practiced, the methods by which research is performed, and how healthcare entities offer critical resources to reach the masses. Many other use cases are only just being uncovered or are not yet even contemplated. This modern approach is happening at the same time patients, health care consumers, research subjects, and even clinicians *themselves* are just beginning to understand and ask for additional privacy protections as well as grasp the implications of how health information can be joined with and used by AI. Knowing the purpose of the AI tool provides the place to start.

The importance of complying with current regulations, along with the need for continued examination of future protections will remain a robust focus in healthcare. Clinicians are strongly encouraged to have at minimum a working knowledge of the categories and types of data being acquired, accessed, used, processed, and/or disclosed when engaging with AI. Practitioners and users of AI should take care to assess and account for the risks, and when applicable collaborate with the entity designated privacy official or counsel to make certain all laws are prudently followed with respect to the use cases, data types, and overall requirements in the effort to prevent information outflow and potential breach and trust issues.

Risks can be managed through varying techniques. These can include developing vigorous data maintenance, retention and destruction policies and procedures or the implementation of a privacy or AI framework and robust governance structure. Anonymized, fully de-identified, or synthetic data should be considered whenever possible. Privacy by Design principles are a preemptive approach to mitigating risk. AI can be successful when innovation is effectively balanced with data privacy rights, fair information practices, transparency, and use of authorization or consent as applicable.

References

1. Taylor P. Volume of data/information created, captured, copied, and consumed worldwide from 2010 to 2020, with forecasts from 2021 to 2025. Statista. Updated November 16, 2023. https://www.statista.com/statistics/871513/worldwide-data-created/#statisticContainer. Accessed 4 May 2024.
2. Ataman A. Data quality in AI: challenges, importance & best practices in '24. AI Multiple Research. Updated January 3, 2024. https://research.aimultiple.com/data-quality-ai/. Accessed 4 May 2024.
3. Albert Henry T. Patients want privacy, accountability for how their health data is used. American Medical Association. Updated August 15, 2022. https://www.ama-assn.org/delivering-care/patient-support-advocacy/patients-want-privacy-accountability-how-their-health-data. Accessed 5 May 2024.
4. Tyson A, Pasquini G, Spencer A, Funk C. 60% of Americans would be uncomfortable with provider relying on AI in their own health care. Pew Research Center. Updated February 22, 2023. https://www.pewresearch.org/science/2023/02/22/60-of-americans-would-be-uncomfortable-with-provider-relying-on-ai-in-their-own-health-care/. Accessed 5 May 2024.

5. Asan O, Bayrak AE, Choudhury A. Artificial intelligence and human trust in healthcare: focus on clinicians. J Med Internet Res. 2020;22(6):e15154.
6. Sterling E, Siira E, Nilsen P, Svedberg P, Nygren J. Implementing AI in healthcare-the relevance of trust: a scoping review. Front Health Serv. 2023;3:1211150.
7. United States Cybersecurity and Infrastructure Security Agency. Critical infrastructure sectors. United States Cybersecurity and Infrastructure Security Agency Critical Infrastructure Security and Resilience. https://www.cisa.gov/topics/critical-infrastructure-security-and-resilience/critical-infrastructure-sectors. Accessed 6 May 2024.
8. United States Department of Health and Human Services. Code of Federal Regulations. https://www.govinfo.gov/content/pkg/CFR-2023-title45-vol2/pdf/CFR-2023-title45-vol2-part164.pdf. Accessed 6 May 2024.
9. United States Department of Health and Human Services. Summary of HIPAA Privacy Rule. https://www.hhs.gov/hipaa/for-professionals/privacy/laws-regulations/index.html. Accessed 6 May 2024.
10. Kim HL, Hyun SS. The future of medical tourism for individuals' health and well-being: a case study of the relationship improvement between the UAE (United Arab Emirates) and South Korea. Int J Environ Res Public Health. 2022;19(9):5735.
11. Folks A. US state privacy legislation tracker. International Association of Privacy Professionals. Updated May 6, 2024. https://iapp.org/resources/article/us-state-privacy-legislation-tracker/. Accessed 7 May 2024.
12. Davis O, Stauss D. A look at proposed US state private sector AI legislation. International Association of Privacy Professionals. Updated February 24, 2024. https://iapp.org/news/a/a--look-at-proposed-u-s-state-private-sector-ai-legislation/. Accessed 7 May 2024.
13. General Data Protection Regulation. Complete guide to GDPR compliance. https://gdprinfo.eu/. Accessed 7 May 2024.
14. Andrews C. European parliament approves landmark AI act, looks ahead to implementation. International Association of Privacy Professionals. Updated March 13, 2024. https://iapp.org/news/a/with-eu-ai-act-on-the-books-lawmakers-look-ahead/. Accessed 7 May 2024.
15. The White House. Fact sheet: President Biden issues executive order on safe, secure, and trustworthy artificial intelligence. Published October 30, 2023. https://www.whitehouse.gov/briefing-room/statements-releases/2023/10/30/fact-sheet-president-biden-issues-executive-order-on-safe-secure-and-trustworthy-artificial-intelligence/. Accessed 7 May 2024.
16. American Medical Association Code of Medical Ethics. 3.1.1 Privacy in Health Care. https://code-medical-ethics.ama-assn.org/sites/amacoedb/files/2022-08/3.1.1.pdf. Accessed 11 May 2024.
17. Nass S, Levit L, Gostin L. Beyond the HIPAA privacy rule: enhancing privacy, improving health through research. In: Institute of Medicine (US) Committee on Health Research and the Privacy of Health Information: The HIPAA Privacy Rule. Washington, DC: National Academy of Sciences Press; 2009. p. 75–110.
18. The Office of the National Coordinator for Health Information Technology. Chapter 4: Integrating privacy and security into your practice. In: Guide to privacy and security of health information. https://www.healthit.gov/sites/default/files/pdf/privacy/privacy_and_security_chapter4.pdf. Accessed 11 May 2024.
19. Granado A, Sottara D, Singh R, Murcko A, Soni H, Tang T, et al. Pilot evaluation of sensitive data segmentation technology for privacy. Int J Med Inform. 2020;138:1–9.
20. White R, Horvitz E. From web search to healthcare utilization: privacy-sensitive studies from mobile data. J Am Med Inform Assoc. 2013;20(1):61–8.
21. Dhar A, Fera B, Korenda L. Can GenAI help make health care affordable? Consumers think so. Deloitte. Updated November 16, 2023. https://www2.deloitte.com/us/en/blog/health-care-blog/2023/can-gen-ai-help-make-health-care-affordable-consumers-think-so.html. Accessed 12 May 2024.
22. Andreotta AJ, Kirkham N, Rizzi M. AI, big data, and the future of consent. AI & Soc. 2022;37(4):1715–28.

23. Senarath A, Asanka Gamagedara Arachchilage N. A data minimization model for embedding privacy into software systems. Comput Secur. 2019;87:1–17.
24. Lee HP, Yang YJ, Serban Von Davier T, Forlizzi J, Das S. Deepfakes, phrenology, surveillance, and more! A taxonomy of AI privacy risks. In: CHI '24: Proceedings of the CHI conference on human factors in computing systems, vol. 775; 2024. p. 1–19.
25. Moraes HB, Previtali MB. Shaping the future: a dynamic taxonomy for AI privacy risks. International Association of Privacy Professionals. Updated January 17, 2024. https://iapp.org/news/a/shaping-the-future-a-dynamic-taxonomy-for-ai-privacy-risks. Accessed 19 May 2024.
26. Blackman R, Ammanath B. Building transparency into AI projects. Harvard Business Review. Updated June 20, 2022. https://hbr.org/2022/06/building-transparency-into-ai-projects. Accessed 26 May 2024.
27. Ambigavathi M, Sridharan D. Big data analytics in healthcare. In: Tenth International Conference on Advanced Computing (ICoAC); 2018. p. 269–76.
28. Federal Privacy Council. Fair Information Practice Principles (FIPPs). https://www.fpc.gov/resources/fipps/. Accessed 28 May 2024.
29. National Institute of Standards and Technology. NIST Privacy Framework: A Tool for Improving Privacy Through Enterprise Risk Management, Version 1.0. https://nvlpubs.nist.gov/nistpubs/CSWP/NIST.CSWP.01162020.pdf. Accessed 29 May 2024.
30. National Institute of Standards and Technology. Artificial Intelligence Risk Management Framework (AI RMF 1.0). https://nvlpubs.nist.gov/nistpubs/ai/NIST.AI.100-1.pdf. Accessed 29 May 2024.
31. Office of the Information and Privacy Commissioner of Ontario. Privacy by Design Seven Foundation Principles. https://www.ipc.on.ca/sites/default/files/legacy/2018/01/pbd-1.pdf. Accessed 30 May 2024.
32. Eastwood B. What is synthetic data—and how can it help you competitively? MIT Sloan School of Management. Updated January 23, 2023. https://mitsloan.mit.edu/ideas-made-to-matter/what-synthetic-data-and-how-can-it-help-you-competitively. Accessed 31 May 2024.
33. The Organisation for Economic Co-operation and Development. Emerging privacy enhancing technologies: current regulatory and policy approaches. https://www.oecd-ilibrary.org/docserver/bf121be4-en.pdf?expires=1717102612&id=id&accname=ocid177408&checksum=C209FF0642F98B0565081309457639F2. Accessed 30 May 2024.
34. Jordan S, Fontaine C, Hendricks-Sturrup R. Selecting privacy-enhancing technologies for managing health data use. Front Public Health. 2022;10(814163):1–13.

Chapter 13
Cybersecurity Challenges of Digital Health and AI in Healthcare

Alyssa Abo and Shannon Lantzy

Introduction

Cybersecurity is a critical component of patient safety, care delivery, and the functioning of hospitals. U.S. healthcare is in "cyber critical condition." For clinicians, the first-order principle is to care for patients. As a nation, we have inadvertently built a fragile healthcare infrastructure. The aim is to rebuild to a desired state wherein cybersecurity is largely invisible to clinicians, so that they may maintain focus on patient care. Until that end is achieved, physicians must be advocates, open-minded, and collaborators in the process of protecting against and responding to cyber-attacks.

Today, one of the most common cyber attacks on hospitals involve ransomware. A ransomware attack is when criminal actors freeze information systems to hold hospitals hostage for a ransom payment. Most attacks are delivered through malware when employees of healthcare institutions inadvertently click on a link or attachment. This is how a Vermont health system was brought down when a clinician took her laptop on vacation, let her adult daughter check her personal email, her daughter clicked on a link or attachment, and malware infected the computer. When the clinician returned to the hospital 2 weeks later and logged onto the hospital network, the malware instantly spread to the health system's electronic medical record system. This attack cost the hospital over $63 million in expenses and lost revenue (insurance only covered $30 M), caused reversion to paper for a month

A. Abo
Impact1 at Stanford Mussallem Center for Biodesign, Stanford Medicine, Stanford, CA, USA

S. Lantzy (✉)
Shannon Lantzy, LLC, Silver Spring, MD, USA
e-mail: shannon@shannonlantzy.com

T. Adirim (ed.), *Digital Health, AI and Generative AI in Healthcare*,
https://doi.org/10.1007/978-3-031-83526-1_13

while the electronic health record (EHR) was down, and overall recovery from the incident took more than 11 months. Patients were diverted, treatment records were unavailable, and clinicians were stretched extremely thin.

In policy, cyber hygiene is discussed as being the basics for organizations that need to protect their infrastructure. This is a "hand washing" moment. It took 100 years from the discovery of handwashing to preventing laboring mothers' deaths to instilling it as a universal practice. The analogy is apt but for one element: the cyber handwashing of today (e.g., don't click on unknown links, use multi-factor authentication) may change tomorrow. Cybersecurity is a moving target.

As healthcare increasingly relies on digital and cyber-physical systems to deliver essential services, the integration of robust cybersecurity measures has never been more urgent. This chapter explores the multifaceted nature of cybersecurity harms in healthcare settings, the vulnerability of systems crucial to patient care, and practical instruction for the clinician's role in mitigating these risks.

Cyber-attacks in healthcare are not only common but are driven by a diverse array of actors with various motives—from criminally motivated ransomware attacks to potentially catastrophic data corruption through injection attacks. These incidents can cripple critical healthcare infrastructure, from imaging equipment like CTs and MRIs to essential operational systems including EHR and payroll systems. The consequences are varied, including disrupted healthcare services, compromised patient safety, jeopardized medical data privacy, and increased workload for the clinicians left to provide care without digital tools.

The challenges are exacerbated by the interconnectedness of modern healthcare ecosystems. Attacks have been launched through seemingly peripheral entry points such as payroll and revenue cycle systems, demonstrating that weakness in the clinical infrastructure can originate from unexpected dependencies. Moreover, every participant in the healthcare system, from clinicians and administrators to patients themselves, plays a vital role in maintaining cybersecurity.

Healthcare faces unique challenges in cybersecurity. Robust cybersecurity measures in other sectors, such as multi-factor authentication, can slow down clinical workflows. The allure of digital health solutions, offering to bridge clinical gaps and address challenges such as staffing shortages and informational deficits, has introduced complex, interconnected networks that are difficult to secure. Security is often "hidden" and therefore under-developed. The healthcare sector must balance rigorous security measures with the imperative to maintain seamless clinical workflows—an equilibrium that was made tougher by the rapid adoption of EHRs under initiatives like the Meaningful Use program instituted through legislation passed in 2009.

Cybersecurity in healthcare is uniquely challenging, underscored by the sector's rapid digitalization and the critical nature of its services. There are varying roles and responsibilities at every level – from policymakers mandating industry-wide security enhancements, as seen in recent FDA guidance, to the everyday actions of healthcare professionals who can fortify their defenses against cyber threats. Practical guidance is provided on how medical professionals can contribute to safeguarding their systems, emphasizing that our digital defenses are only as strong as their weakest link.

It is important for everyone to appreciate the pervasive risk of cybersecurity threats in healthcare, understand the integral role of every system user, and be equipped with the knowledge to actively participate in protecting their cyber-physical environments. This is not just a matter of policy or technology; it is a fundamental aspect of patient care.

Real Attacks on Hospitals and Health Systems

Attacks can be economically motivated. Some are nation-state attacks [1]. Others may be motivated by personal activism. "Nearly all cyberattacks, and digital data thefts begin the same way - with human error." [2] Below are a few examples that illustrate the types of attacks and their causes, and a small sample of their impacts.

University of Vermont Medical Center [3]

Route of attack: The clinician lent her daughter her work laptop to check personal email.

Impact: Over $63 million in expenses and lost revenue (insurance only covered $30 M), caused reversion to paper for a month while the HER was down, and overall recovery took more than 11 months. Patients were diverted, treatment records were unavailable, and clinicians were stretched extremely thin.

Change Healthcare [4]

Route of attack: UnitedHealth failed to use multi-factor authentication.

Impact: "The Change Healthcare cyberattack is the most significant and consequential incident of its kind against the U.S. healthcare system in history," Rick Pollack, president and CEO of the American Hospital Association, said in a statement. "This attack has made it harder for hospitals to provide patient care, fill prescriptions, submit insurance claims and receive payment for the essential healthcare services they provide." [5].

"Ninety-four percent of hospitals are experiencing a financial impact from the Change Healthcare cyberattack with more than half reporting "significant or serious" impact, according to results from an AHA survey released today. The survey included responses from about 1000 hospitals from March 9 to 12. More than 80% of hospitals said the cyberattack has affected their cash flow, and of those nearly 60% report that the impact to revenue is $1 million per day or more. In addition, the survey found that 74% of hospitals reported impacts to direct patient care as a result of the cyberattack. "[5].

Ascension [6]

Route of attack: Accidental download of malware (presumed phishing).

Impact: "The health system asked patients to bring appointment notes as well as lists of prescriptions or pill bottles, so their providers could call in medication needs. Some hospitals in Indiana, Michigan, Oklahoma, and Tennessee had to divert ambulances during the cyberattack."

Volt Typhoon [7]

While not an attack on a U.S. hospital, a Chinese state-sponsored hacking group is targeting critical infrastructure like our communication, water, and transportation infrastructure. This type of infrastructure could shut down access to water, which is essential for a functioning hospital system.

Because reporting is not yet mandatory for hospitals, the above examples are a small subset of real attacks and possible attack routes. Many anecdotes exist and are often reported in the media. For more up-to-date lists of cyber incidents in healthcare:

- List of attacks causing emergency diversion and impacts: https://thereadable.co/a-list-of-healthcare-cyberattacks-that-disrupted-emergency-services-in-2023/
- List of healthcare data breaches: https://www.healthcaredive.com/news/tracking-healthcare-data-breaches-cybersecurity-hacking-hospitals/696184/

Impacts of Cybersecurity Attacks on Healthcare

"Healthcare is in critical condition." Cybersecurity attacks harm patients, providers, and health systems [8].

Impact on Patients

Cybersecurity breaches in healthcare settings harm patients. Ransomware or nation-state attacks compromise the safety and effectiveness of care delivery, often with severe consequences. A growing body of evidence illustrates the tangible and sometimes devastating impact of cyber incidents on patient outcomes.

At the University of Vermont Medical Center (mentioned above), a ransomware attack crippled systems for nearly a month, with full recovery requiring over 11 months. This disruption severely affected patient care, delaying chemotherapy treatments, and forcing the rescheduling of critical patient appointments and procedures. The inability to access EHR and diagnostic services compromised the timely and effective treatment of patients, underlining the direct link between cybersecurity and patient safety [9].

In another alarming incident, a baby in Illinois suffered due to delayed medical procedures following a cyberattack. The attack disrupted the systems necessary for timely diagnostic tests and medical interventions. This delay highlights a critical issue: when cyber intrusions cause medical devices and support systems to go offline, the most vulnerable patients can experience immediate and life-threatening consequences [10].

Disruptions from cybersecurity incidents are not isolated to the targeted facility; they often have a cascading effect on surrounding healthcare centers [11, 12]. When one hospital diverts its emergency services, nearby facilities can become overwhelmed, further straining resources and compromising patient care across a region.

These examples underline the necessity of robust cybersecurity protocols and continuous vigilance. As healthcare continues to integrate advanced technologies, the potential for cyber-induced patient harm escalates, making the protection of healthcare systems an imperative component of patient safety.

Impact on Providers

Cyber-attacks in healthcare settings exacerbate the challenges already faced by providers, particularly those who are already at high risk of burnout. When systems go down, the workload on healthcare staff increases dramatically; simple tasks that were once automated or streamlined through digital systems now require manual intervention. For example, instead of an online order to the pharmacy, an clinicians will have to handwrite orders and staff might have to physically go in person to retrieve medications. This increased burden acts as a force divider, stretching thin resources even thinner and amplifying the stress on an already overtaxed workforce.

The reliance on digital tools and AI in modern healthcare has streamlined many processes but also created a dependency that becomes acutely problematic during cyber-attacks. With systems down, healthcare providers might struggle with tasks they used to manage automatically, such as recalling specific medication dosages or formulations—knowledge that is less readily accessible due to the reduced personal reliance on memory and manual processes. A nurses' union representative from Ascension highlighted the severity of the situation, noting how these disruptions not only increase operational burdens but also significantly impact the quality of patient care, as critical information is not as readily available or accurate.

Impact on Health Systems and Hospitals

Hospitals, already operating under significant operational burdens and tight financial margins, face compounded challenges when dealing with cybersecurity threats. The costs associated with strengthening cyber defenses and responding to attacks can be substantial, diverting scarce resources away from patient care and other critical operations. This financial strain is exacerbated during actual cyber incidents, which can cripple hospital operations and lead to severe revenue disruptions. For instance, Change Healthcare experienced a staggering 12 days without revenue due to a cyberattack, illustrating the profound economic impact these events can have on healthcare organizations.

Moreover, the vulnerability of hospitals to cyber threats can result in closure. At least one hospital has cited cyberattacks as a contributing factor in their decision to close. This can be particularly devastating for communities with critical access hospitals, which serve vital needs in rural areas but are closing at an alarming rate. These facilities are often less equipped to handle the dual challenges of cybersecurity and operational sustainability compared to larger urban hospitals with more resources. The closure of these essential hospitals not only deprives rural communities of immediate healthcare access but also underscores the broader systemic vulnerabilities in healthcare infrastructure that are exacerbated by cyber threats.

Types of Threats, Types of Harm

Attacks come through varied channels, can be combined together, and can change at any moment. Five areas of threat:

- Social Engineering (e.g., phishing), where attackers gain sensitive data or credentials by posing as a legitimate communication
- Ransomware, where malicious software is downloaded to a computer then spreads through a network and locks up a system or data, holding it hostage
- Loss of equipment or theft, where data or credentials on hardware (e.g., discs, thumb drives, laptops, etc.) are found or stolen
- Insider or accidental data loss, where legitimate users on the network either purposefully or accidentally cause system downtime or data loss
- Attacks against network-connected medical devices, where the network-connected device can be used to perform unintended operations (either physically or on the network)

Ransomware is the most common and frequently experienced cyber incident reported in the news. Some other attacks may never be detected or may be detected years later. Individuals may refer to HHS publications and materials for up-to-date information on attacks [13]. HHS' website provides training resources on each of these five threats, including easy-to-use one-page job aids (see example in the image below) as well as training videos and PowerPoint presentations.

What is Social Engineering?

Social engineering is a form of psychological manipulation that tricks users into making security mistakes or giving away sensitive information. It relies on human error, instead of vulnerabilities in software and operating systems, by exploiting human emotions.

Steps to take

Review this checklist and follow each recommendation.

If you answer 'Yes' to any of these, **please act immediately.**

Action—Report

Contact your IT administrator, practice manager or immediate supervisor to report this email. Add their name and number to this sheet for reference.

Phishing Checklist

HHS 405(d) Knowledge on Demand

- ☐ Don't recognize the sender?
- ☐ Not expecting an attachment or email?
- ☐ Does 'From' address match message?
- ☐ Does this invoke a sense of urgency?
- ☐ Don't recognize the destination URL
- ☐ Is this standard internal procedure for IT issues?
- ☐ Is this website secure? (https://)
- ☐ Is this email asking for your login credentials?
- ☐ Is there bad grammar or spelling?
- ☐ Is the greeting/signature generic or lack contact info?

Reporting

Report to:

Contact Info:

For more resources and to learn more about how you can protect your patients from cyber threats, check out the *Health Industry Cybersecurity Practices: Managing Threats and Protecting Patients (HICP)* publication at 405d.hhs.gov.

What you need to know about Ransomware:

Ransomware poses a threat to you and your device. What makes this form of malware so unique is the word "ransom". Ransomware is extortion software that can lock your computer and then demand a ransom for its release.

Cybersecurity threats to health care organizations and patient safety are real. Information technology, which provides critical life-saving functions, consists of connected and networked systems and leverages wireless technologies, leaving such systems more vulnerable to cyber-attack.

Steps to take

Review the list of best practices and follow each recommendation.

Action—Report

Contact your IT administrator, practice manager, or immediate supervisor. Any suspicious activity on your system? Add their name and number to this sheet for reference.

Quick action in this case is imperative. This threat is real!

Threat Quick Tips

HHS 405(d) Knowledge on Demand

Most ransomware attacks are sent in phishing campaign emails. These messages ask you to either open an attachment or click on an embedded link.

- ☑ **Stay alert** when any email prompts you to enter your credentials.
- ☑ **Be cautious** before clicking any links in an email. Look at the sender address and hover over the URL.
- ☑ As a proactive measure, **check to see** whether the computer and network to which you are connected have the proper intrusion prevention system or software in place.
- ☑ Due to the severity and time sensitivity of ransomware attacks, **seek out professional IT security (or a similar point of contact)** help when you think your computer is infected with ransomware.

Reporting

Report to:

Contact Info:

For more resources and to learn more about how you can protect your patients from cyber threats, check out the *Health Industry Cybersecurity Practices: Managing Threats and Protecting Patients (HICP)* publication at 405d.hhs.gov.

Types of cybersecurity harm include loss of **confidentiality** (data exposure), loss of **integrity** (data or credentials has been manipulated or otherwise cannot be authenticated), or loss of **availability** (system is down). This is known as the CIA triad. Any of the types of threat listed above can cause a loss of CIA.

Clinician's Role: Prevention, Response, and Supporting Patients

In an era where digital health and artificial intelligence (AI) systems are integral to healthcare, safeguarding these technologies against cybersecurity threats is crucial. The solutions to this challenge must arise from all levels of our healthcare infrastructure, encompassing national trade and defense policy, regulatory frameworks, technology producers, medical device companies, health systems, providers, and patients. However, clinicians play a particularly pivotal role in this multifaceted defense strategy.

Responsibilities: The Collective Effort: A Multi-Level Approach

National Trade, Critical Infrastructure, and Defense Policy

At the national level, trade and defense policies must prioritize cybersecurity in healthcare. This involves setting stringent import standards for medical devices and digital health tools and ensuring that they meet rigorous cybersecurity benchmarks. Additionally, fostering international cooperation on cybersecurity can help create a global standard, reducing vulnerabilities across borders.

Health Regulators

In 2024, there were several cybersecurity initiatives under consideration by HHS and Congress [14] and the National Cybersecurity Strategy Implementation Plan [15] was released by the Biden White House. Regulatory bodies like the FDA and other health authorities need to enforce and update national cybersecurity guidelines for digital health technologies. They should mandate comprehensive security assessments before approving new devices and periodically re-evaluate existing technologies. Robust regulatory oversight ensures that manufacturers and healthcare providers adhere to best practices in cybersecurity.

Technology Producers and MedTech Companies

Manufacturers of digital health technologies must prioritize security by design. This means integrating cybersecurity measures from the initial design phase through the end of the product's lifecycle. Technology producers should collaborate closely with healthcare experts in Cybersecurity to understand and address specific security needs, ensuring their products are resilient against emerging threats.

Health Systems

Healthcare systems and institutions must implement strong cybersecurity policies and protocols. This includes regular vulnerability assessments, timely software updates, and continuous monitoring for potential breaches. Health systems should also invest in advanced cybersecurity infrastructure and foster a culture of security awareness among all employees. Specific cybersecurity performance goals for hospitals are published by HHS and (as of 2024), there is legislation under development to make these mandatory.

Clinicians: The Frontline Defenders

While systemic efforts are essential, clinicians are the frontline defenders in protecting digital health and AI systems. Their direct interaction with these technologies places them in a unique position to identify vulnerabilities and implement preventive measures.

Prevention

Continuous Education and Training

Clinicians must receive ongoing training in cybersecurity best practices. Given the rapid evolution of cyber threats, it is crucial for healthcare providers to stay updated and undergo 'cyber-hygiene' exercises with the latest prevention strategies [16]. Regular refresher courses, mandatory training, and hands-on exercises can enhance their ability to recognize and respond to potential threats. Online resources such as "Cybersecurity for the Clinician" provide an overview and introduction for clinicians [17].

Securing User Accounts

Several practical steps can significantly bolster the security of digital health systems:

- **Multi-Factor Authentication (MFA):** Clinicians should use MFA to add an extra layer of security, making it more difficult for unauthorized users to access sensitive systems.

- **Strong Password Practices:** Changing factory default passwords and using strong, unique passwords for different systems can prevent unauthorized access. Hospitals often require staff to update passwords at given intervals of time. Password memorization is a challenge; adopting password managers and biometrics identification are alternatives.
- **Timely Software Updates:** Ensuring that all devices and systems are regularly patched and updated can mitigate vulnerabilities, including any device that interacts on the hospital's networks (i.e., laptops, phones).
- **Never lend your device to someone else who isn't authorized:** The Vermont ransomware attack originated from a clinical allowing her adult daughter to check her personal email on the work laptop during a vacation. One-click by her daughter brought the system to a halt for days, and recovery took 11 months.
- **Personal commitment and discipline:** Follow the best practices in this list, and those in training courses provided by the clinician's institution, even when it is inconvenient. If cybersecurity measures prevent quality clinical care, report it to the appropriate leader (e.g., report it as an adverse event for medical devices).

Phishing remains a significant threat, often targeting healthcare providers as entry points into larger systems. Regular phishing training for clinicians is improving, but continuous vigilance is necessary. Nearly 1 in 7 simulated phishing events are successful [18]. By being aware of common phishing tactics and knowing how to respond, clinicians can prevent many cyber-attacks from gaining a foothold.

Communication and Collaboration

Effective communication between clinicians and technology developers is vital. Clinicians should actively communicate their usability needs and security concerns to industry collaborators, ensuring that the products they evaluate are both effective and secure. They should also participate in cybersecurity discussions within their institutions, contributing to policymaking and risk assessment processes.

Influencing Technology Adoption

Clinicians have significant influence over the adoption of new medical technologies. It is often second nature to inquire about FDA status and reimbursement strategies. In addition to regulatory and financial considerations, they should include cybersecurity considerations in their decision-making process, asking proactive critical questions such as:

- How is the technology secured by design?
- How does the technology mitigate cybersecurity risks?

- What are the procedures for maintaining security throughout the technology's lifecycle?
- What measures are in place to protect patient data and comply with privacy regulations?
- How will the technology perform during an attack?

By continuously seeking to improve their cybersecurity knowledge and practices, clinicians can significantly contribute to the overall security of digital health and AI systems. By asking these questions, clinicians can better vet the technologies that are presented to them.

Response: Plans for Supporting Patients During and After Cyber Attacks

Clinicians and their trade organizations can also play a crucial role in helping patients navigate the complexities of digital health technologies [19, 20]. This includes:

- **Education:** Teaching patients how to use their medical devices securely, such as diabetes management tools, CPAP machines, and pacemakers.
- **Guidance:** Providing clear instructions on how to maintain device security, such as recognizing phishing attempts and avoiding unsecured networks.

As healthcare increasingly moves into the home setting, ensuring that patients understand and implement cybersecurity practices is essential for protecting their health data and personal information.

Training and Information Resources for Clinicians and Other Healthcare Personnel

- Knowledge on Demand is the 405(d) Program's free cybersecurity education platform. It includes multiple levels of delivery methodologies designed to reach the varied size healthcare facilities across the country. This platform includes cybersecurity awareness trainings that align with the top 5 cybersecurity threats outlined in the landmark 405(d) Health Industry Cybersecurity Practices publication [21].
- The Health Sector Coordinating Council Cybersecurity Working Group provides a clinician training series of videos that provides a comprehensive view of the risks of their technology to cybersecurity incidents [22].

- I Am The Cavalry, an organization of volunteers globally with diverse backgrounds and a range of expertise across technology, law, and public policy provides a “Hippocratic Oath for Connected Medical Devices” that provides information about maintaining cyber safety [23].
- Tabletop Exercises and scenario-based training clarify an institution or system’s vulnerabilities and support determining processes for reacting to cybersecurity incidents. An example of such a tabletop exercise is described in an Academic Medicine article [24].

Conclusion

Protecting digital health and AI systems in healthcare requires a comprehensive, multi-level approach. While national policies, regulatory frameworks, and technological innovations are critical, clinicians play a central role in this defense strategy. In recent years, the federal government has been extremely concerned about the escalation of cybersecurity incidents on healthcare and they have been proposing best practices and mandates that healthcare personnel and leaders must be aware of and be prepared to institute [14].

Through education, proactive security measures, effective communication, and patient support, clinicians can help safeguard the technologies transforming healthcare, ensuring they remain secure and beneficial for all.

Acknowledgments Cofounders of CyberMed (Josh Corman, Beau Woods, Christian Dameff, Jeff Tully) and the leaders of the Health Sector Coordinating Council Cybersecurity Working Group for their volunteer time and effort for the whole industry. Josh Corman for his guidance on this chapter and for his focus on protecting patients and providers.

References

1. Cybersecurity and Infrastructure Security Agency. PRC State-Sponsored Actors Compromise and Maintain Persistent Access to U.S. Critical Infrastructure. Cybersecurity Advisory AA24-038A. Published February 7, 2024. https://www.cisa.gov/news-events/cybersecurity-advisories/aa24-038a. Accessed 22 June 2024.
2. America’s Healthcare Networks Are Under Attack. Healthcare dive. Published April 4, 2024. https://www.healthcaredive.com/spons/americas-healthcare-networks-are-under-attack/715747/. Accessed 22 June 2024.
3. Gentile D. UVM Medical Center Cyber Attack. Vermont House Energy and Technology Committee. Published March 31, 2022. https://legislature.vermont.gov/Documents/2022/WorkGroups/House%20Energy%20and%20Technology/Technology/Cybersecurity/W~Douglas%20Gentile~UVM%20Medical%20Center%20Cyber%20Attack~3-31-2022.pdf. Accessed 29 Sept 2024.
4. House Committee on Energy and Commerce. What we learned: change healthcare cyber attack. Published May 3, 2024. https://energycommerce.house.gov/posts/what-we-learned-change-healthcare-cyber-attack. Accessed 22 June 2024.

5. Blum K, Burns J. The impact of the change healthcare cyberattack: what to know. Association of Health Care Journalists. Published April 5, 2024. https://healthjournalism.org/blog/2024/04/the-impact-of-the-change-healthcare-cyberattack-what-to-know/. Accessed 22 June 2024.
6. Jones C. How did the cyberattack on major hospital system ascension happen? Milwaukee Journal Sentinel. Published June 13, 2024. https://www.jsonline.com/story/money/business/2024/06/13/how-did-the-cyberattack-on-major-hospital-system-ascension-happen/74084483007/. Accessed 22 June 2024.
7. University of Maryland, Baltimore County. What is Volt Typhoon? A cybersecurity expert explains the Chinese hackers targeting U.S. critical infrastructure. Published June 8, 2023. https://umbc.edu/stories/what-is-volt-typhoon-a-cybersecurity-expert-explains-the-chinese-hackers-targeting-us-critical-infrastructure/. Accessed 29 Sept 2024.
8. Healthcare IT News. Pandemic stress, cyberattacks are compounding the degradation of care delivery. Published January 6, 2021. https://www.healthcareitnews.com/news/pandemic-stress-cyberattacks-are-compounding-degradation-care-delivery. Accessed 29 Sept 2024.
9. O'Donnell B, Stempniak M. Cyberattacks disrupting patient care at alarming rate, report finds. Healthcare Dive. October 29, 2020. https://www.healthcaredive.com/news/cyberattacks-hospitals-disrupt-operations-patient-care-Ponemon/631439/. Accessed 26 June 2024.
10. Jena AB, Mann NC, Wedlund LN, Olenski A. Delays in emergency care and mortality during major U.S. marathons. N Engl J Med. 2017;376(15):1441–50.
11. Dameff C, Tully J, Chan TC, Castillo EM, Savage S, Maysent P, et al. Effectiveness of a digital mental health intervention in reducing symptoms of depression: a randomized clinical trial. JAMA Netw Open. 2023;6(4):e43066. https://jamanetwork.com/journals/jamanetworkopen/article-abstract/2804585. Accessed 22 June 2024
12. The Joint Commission. Sentinel Event Alert 67: Cybersecurity. Published July 26, 2023. https://www.jointcommission.org/-/media/tjc/newsletters/sea-67-cybersecurity-7-26-23-final.pdf. Accessed 22 June 2024.
13. HHS 405(d) Program. The five current threats. https://405d.hhs.gov/kod/five-threats. Accessed 22 June 2024.
14. College of Healthcare Information Management Executives (CHIME). Cybersecurity incentives and penalties under consideration. https://chimecentral.org/content/cheat-sheet-cybersecurity-incentives-and-penalties-under-consideration. Accessed 22 June 2024.
15. U.S. Government. National Cybersecurity Strategy Implementation Plan Version 2. Washington, DC: The White House; 2024. https://www.whitehouse.gov/wp-content/uploads/2024/05/NCSIP-Version-2-FINAL-May-2024.pdf. Accessed 22 June 2024.
16. Priestman W, Anstis T, Sebire IG, Sridharan S, Sebire NJ. Phishing in healthcare organisations: threats, mitigation and approaches. BMJ Health Care Inform. 2019;26(1):e100031.
17. Health Sector Coordinating Council. CyberClinician videos. https://healthsectorcouncil.org/cyberclinicianvideos/. Accessed 22 June 2024.
18. Gordon WJ, Wright A, Aiyagari R, Corbo L, Glynn RJ, Kadakia J, et al. Assessment of employee susceptibility to phishing attacks at US health care institutions. JAMA Netw Open. 2019;2(3):e190393. https://pubmed.ncbi.nlm.nih.gov/30848810/. Accessed 22 June 2024.
19. Sullivan N, Tully J, Dameff C, Opara C, Snead M, Selzer J. A national survey of hospital cyber attack emergency operation preparedness. Disaster Med Public Health Prep. 2023;17:e363. https://www.cambridge.org/core/journals/disaster-medicine-and-public-health-preparedness/article/national-survey-of-hospital-cyber-attack-emergency-operation-preparedness/2091081A25D641D42D915C1F0E823CC2. Accessed 22 June 2024
20. Preparedness and Response Playbook. MITRE. Published November 14, 2022. https://www.mitre.org/news-insights/publication/medical-device-cybersecurity-regional-incident-preparedness-and-response. Accessed 22 June 2024.
21. U.S. Department of Health and Human Services. Health Care Sector Cybersecurity Coordination Center: Cybersecurity Considerations for the Health Care Sector. Published December 2023. https://aspr.hhs.gov/cyber/Documents/Health-Care-Sector-Cybersecurity-Dec2023-508.pdf. Accessed 29 Sept 2024.

22. Health Sector Coordinating Council. Cyber clinician videos. https://healthsectorcouncil.org/cyberclinicianvideos/. Accessed 29 Sept 2024.
23. I Am the Cavalry. The Hippocratic Oath for connected medical devices. https://iamthecavalry.org/issues/medical/oath/. Accessed 29 Sept 2024.
24. Wells C, Krutzik S, Miller R, Kharrazi H. Cybersecurity challenges and the academic health center: preparing for future threats. Acad Med. 2021;96(6):796–800. https://doi.org/10.1097/ACM.0000000000004073. https://journals.lww.com/academicmedicine/abstract/2021/06000/cybersecurity_challenges_and_the_academic_health.39.aspx. Accessed 29 Sept 2024.

Chapter 14
U.S. and Global Regulatory Frameworks For AI in Healthcare

Terry Adirim and Rashmi Rao

Introduction

Artificial Intelligence (AI) in healthcare is evolving at an unprecedented rate, offering promising innovative solutions that were previously unimaginable. From machine learning algorithms predicting patient outcomes to AI-driven ambient dictation of medical encounters, these technologies are revolutionizing the field. However, without appropriate regulatory frameworks, the deployment of AI in healthcare can pose significant risks. High-profile cases, such as flawed AI algorithms leading to misdiagnoses or biased AI systems exacerbating health disparities, highlight the potential dangers of unregulated AI use. Fairness, transparency and accountability in AI algorithms and large language models are why guardrails, established through regulation, are critical in ensuring responsible development, deployment, and use of AI.

The necessity for regulatory frameworks lies in ensuring the safety, efficacy, and ethical deployment of AI in healthcare. These frameworks provide guidelines and standards for the development, testing, and implementation of AI technologies, safeguarding patient welfare and promoting trust in AI innovations. Moreover, as AI continues to evolve, regulatory practices must be continuously updated to address new challenges and integrate the latest advancements in the field.

Many countries and regional coalitions are establishing regulatory approaches, including the United States, European Union, and the Asia-Pacific region. Comparing these emerging frameworks highlighting differences and similarities, offers insights into how varying regulations impact AI healthcare technologies [1].

T. Adirim (✉)
Departments of Pediatrics and Preventive Medicine and Biostatistics,
Uniformed Services University of the Health Sciences, Bethesda, MD, USA

R. Rao
University of Washington, Engineering Innovation in Health (EIH), Sammamish, WA, USA

T. Adirim (ed.), *Digital Health, AI and Generative AI in Healthcare*,
https://doi.org/10.1007/978-3-031-83526-1_14

Clinician end users and patients are and will continue to be impacted by evolving laws and regulations. Chapter 12 covers laws and regulations governing health data. This chapter discusses the regulatory landscape for AI in healthcare, the agencies that enforce regulations and emerging regulatory frameworks in the U.S. and select countries that have implications for the future of AI technology.

U.S. Current Laws and Regulations

In the U.S., the regulatory framework for artificial intelligence (AI) in healthcare primarily falls under the oversight of the Food and Drug Administration (FDA). The FDA plays a pivotal role in regulating AI and machine learning (ML) technologies', particularly those classified as Software as a Medical Device (SaMD). In 2021, the FDA released its Artificial Intelligence/Machine Learning-Based Software as a Medical Device Action Plan that outlines the FDA's current and future activities for regulating AI and machine learning (ML) systems [2]. It emphasizes the importance of a "predetermined change control plan" to manage the evolving nature of AI models, allowing manufacturers to specify anticipated algorithm changes without undergoing a full regulatory review for each iteration. This approach is designed to address the challenges posed by continuously learning algorithms that adapt based on new data inputs over time.

The FDA's Center for Devices and Radiological Health (CDRH) is the part of the FDA responsible for regulating AI that are designated Software as a Medical Device (SaMD). The FDA's current regulatory approach is a four-pronged approach including (i) assuring quality systems and good machine learning practices (GMLP), (ii) initial premarket assurance of safety and effectiveness, (iii) instituting an approach for modifications after initial review with an established SaMD pre-specifications and algorithm change protocols and (iv) transparency and real-world performance monitoring of AI/ML- based SaMD. The FDA established risk-based classifications of medical devices (Class I, II, and III), depending on their intended use and potential risks to patients. AI systems intended for diagnosis, treatment recommendations, or patient management are typically classified under the higher-risk categories (Class II or III), requiring premarket approval or clearance through pathways such as the 510(k) premarket notification or premarket approval (PMA) [3].

The FDA also introduced the Digital Health Innovation Action Plan and launched the Digital Health Software Precertification (Pre-Cert) Pilot Program, in 2022, which aims to create a more streamlined and efficient regulatory pathway for digital health technologies, including AI tools [4]. The FDA's evolving regulatory approach seeks to balance innovation and patient safety, ensuring that AI/ML-based medical devices can adapt to technological advancements while maintaining high standards of care. Changes in federal leadership will determine future approaches to regulation.

Health Insurance Portability and Accountability Act (HIPAA)

As discussed in Chapter 12, the Health Insurance Portability and Accountability Act (HIPAA), enacted in 1996, is a U.S. law safeguarding an individual's medical information. Specifically, HIPAA sets standards to ensure that personal health information (PHI) is kept confidential and secure, which is especially relevant for AI systems that handle vast amounts of patient data [5]. The HIPAA Privacy Rule and Security Rule are two distinct but related regulations emanating from the HIPAA law that mandates covered entities establish administrative, physical, and technical safeguards to ensure the confidentiality, integrity, and security of PHI. The Office for Civil Rights within the U.S. Department of Health and Human Services enforces HIPAA's rules [6]. The emergence of AI systems that use patient data have spurred discussions about the adequacy of HIPAA in addressing new privacy concerns related to AI, leading to proposals for more stringent data protection regulations. For instance, some legislative efforts are focusing on creating enhanced privacy laws similar to the European General Data Protection Regulation (GDPR) (described later in this chapter) to safeguard patients' personal information as AI adoption increases in the U.S. healthcare sector. Chapter 12 gives a more detailed description of the HIPAA rule and how it applies to AI in healthcare.

International Standards

The International Organization for Standardization (ISO) is an independent, non-governmental international organization that develops and publishes standards to ensure quality, safety, efficiency, and interoperability across various industries, including healthcare [7]. ISO standards are created by experts from around the world who collaborate to establish best practices, which are then adopted by countries and industries to improve systems, processes, and products. In healthcare, ISO standards cover areas such as medical devices, health informatics, quality management systems, and risk management, all aimed at promoting patient safety and improving the quality of care [8].

The United States is an active member of the ISO and participates in the development of ISO standards through the American National Standards Institute (ANSI), which is the official U.S. representative to ISO. While ISO standards are not legally binding in the U.S., many industries, including healthcare, voluntarily adopt them as part of their best practices [9]. Additionally, certain ISO standards, such as ISO 13485 for medical devices, are often used in conjunction with U.S. regulations, including those enforced by the FDA. For instance, compliance with ISO standards may be considered beneficial or required in the process of gaining FDA approval for medical devices.

The ISO has established several standards relevant to healthcare, particularly in the realm of medical devices, health informatics, and quality management systems. Key among these is the aforementioned ISO 13485, which outlines requirements for a quality management system specific to medical devices, ensuring that organizations consistently meet regulatory requirements and produce safe, effective products [8]. Another important standard is ISO 14971, which provides guidelines for the application of risk management to medical devices. In the realm of health informatics, ISO/IEC 27799 offers guidelines for the protection of personal health information in healthcare organizations, complementing security and privacy standards. Pending changes include increased focus on AI in healthcare, with ongoing discussions regarding a new standard (ISO/IEC 23894), which aims to address the governance and risk management of AI systems in healthcare [10]. This emerging standard is expected to provide a framework for the safe, effective, and ethical use of AI powered technologies, helping harmonize global practices as AI becomes more integrated into clinical environments. These evolving standards will play a critical role in ensuring AI-driven solutions are implemented with safety and privacy in mind.

Although the U.S. may not enforce all ISO standards as mandatory, they are widely recognized and influential in setting benchmarks for quality and safety in healthcare, and many organizations choose to adhere to them to ensure compliance with global best practices.

Global Regulatory Frameworks for AI in Healthcare

The use of AI in general and specifically for healthcare has been a global concern. As discussed earlier in this chapter, the United States had taken some steps to regulate AI in healthcare. Other nations' governing bodies have also been working on regulatory frameworks for AI and some, such as the European Union, have made significant progress in putting guardrails around AI use [11]. However, there is no one global body responsible for regulating AI in healthcare.

European Union (EU)

In 2024, the EU introduced a robust risk framework for AI, the EU AI Act. Any AI system being marked in the EU must comply with this Act, which specifies risk-based requirements for high-risk AI systems, mandates establishment of a risk management system, technical documentation, post-market monitoring and transparency. This framework applies to AI systems across the health spectrum with the goal of mitigating potentially harmful effects of AI while also allowing these new technologies to be implemented to benefit patient outcomes [12]. Other aspects of the EU regulatory framework include:

- **General Data Protection Regulation (GDPR):** Similar to the U.S. HIPAA law, GDPR focuses on protecting the privacy of personal data, emphasizing data minimization, purpose limitation, and consent. It also grants individuals rights over their data and mandates stringent security measures [13].

- **Medical Device Regulation (MDR) and the In Vitro Diagnostic Medical Devices Regulation (IVDR):** Regulates AI-based medical devices, ensuring devices perform consistently for its intended purpose and complies with safety and performance through classification, conformity assessments, post-market surveillance, and transparency requirements [14].
- **EMA Guidelines on AI in Drug Development:** Addresses drug discovery through the use of AI in clinical trials, encouraging innovation while focusing on safety, ethics, and collaboration between regulators, industry, and academia [15].

Canada

- **Personal Information Protection and Electronic Documents Act (PIPEDA):** This Canadian law covers the use of personal data, emphasizing consent and accountability. Pending legislation (Bill C-27, the Digital Charter Implementation Act, 2022) proposes enhancements for consumer privacy protection and has three components that includes PIPEDA as well as the Consumer Privacy Protection Act and the Artificial Intelligence and Data Act that together are meant to update Canada's privacy framework [16].
- **Health Canada Regulation of AI-Based Medical Devices:** Ensures AI-based devices undergo pre-market assessments for safety and efficacy. Canada's framework also focuses on transparency, ethics, and reducing bias in AI systems [17].

China

- **Guiding Principles for AI in Healthcare:** Emphasizes innovation and patient safety through policies such as the "New Generation Artificial Intelligence Development Plan" and strong data protection through the Personal Information Protection Law (PIPL) [18].

Japan and South Korea

- **Japan:** AI Health and Medical Strategy focuses on using AI for diagnostics and patient management, with regulatory oversight from the Ministry of Health. Moreover, like other countries, Japan has evolved its regulatory framework to address reviews and approvals for SaMD, digital medical devices, and cybersecurity [19].
- **South Korea:** Similar to the United States, South Korea's Ministry of Food and Drug Safety (MFDS) oversees the development, approval, and monitoring of AI-based medical devices, ensuring data privacy and transparent algorithm performance [20].

Australia and New Zealand

- **Australia's Therapeutic Goods Administration (TGA):** Regulates AI-based medical devices and software with clear pathways for approval, ensuring ongoing safety and efficacy through clinical validation. Australia's TGA provides a comprehensive framework including providing a definition of a medical device, how they are used, how they are regulated and including regulations on large language models (LLMs), synthetic data use, chatbots, and generative AI software [21].
- **New Zealand's MedSafe:** Largely focuses on ethical use and safety for AI in healthcare, with oversight for AI-based medical devices and ensuring transparency in their application [22].

Each of these countries' regulatory frameworks aims to ensure that AI technologies in healthcare are deployed safely, ethically, and effectively, with a strong focus on data protection, transparency, and accountability (Table 14.1).

Impending and Likely U.S. Regulations

Pending and proposed U.S. legislation seek to address the challenges and opportunities presented by AI in healthcare, particularly regarding privacy, data security, and ethical concerns. One significant legislative effort is the Algorithmic Accountability Act, which was first introduced in 2019 and reintroduced in 2022 [23]. This proposed legislation would require companies to evaluate the impacts of their automated decision systems, including AI in healthcare, particularly concerning issues of bias, fairness, and transparency. If passed, healthcare AI developers would be mandated to conduct impact assessments and mitigate risks related to discrimination and privacy violations. Another recent legislative proposal is the Advancing Artificial Intelligence Research Act of 2021, which calls for the establishment of a national AI research task force to promote research and development of trustworthy AI systems, with a particular emphasis on healthcare applications [24]. Neither of these bills passed and therefore would have to be reproposed to become law.

Future Expectations and Challenges

Users of AI in healthcare should expect challenges related to current and upcoming regulations that must adapt to the rapidly evolving nature of AI technologies. One of the main challenges will be managing continuously learning algorithms. Traditional regulatory frameworks are designed for static medical devices, but AI systems, particularly those using machine learning, can evolve over time based on

Table 14.1 Global AI regulatory frameworks and processes

Country/ Region	Regulatory authority	Key regulations	Focus areas
United States	FDA, HIPAA (Health Insurance Portability and Accountability Act)	• FDA: AI/ML-based Software as a Medical Device (SaMD) • HIPAA for data privacy and security	• Pre-market evaluation and post-market surveillance for AI devices • Data protection and privacy • Transparency, safety, and accountability
European Union (EU)	European Medicines Agency (EMA), GDPR (General Data Protection Regulation), MDR (Medical Device Regulation)	• EU AI Act 2024 GDPR for data protection • MDR for AI-based medical devices • EMA for AI in drug development	• Data minimization, purpose limitation, and patient rights • Safety and performance of AI medical devices • Ethical and collaborative AI use
Canada	Health Canada, PIPEDA (Personal Information Protection and Electronic Documents Act)	• AI-based medical devices regulation • PIPEDA for data protection	• Pre-market assessment for AI devices • Ethical AI use, transparency, and reducing bias • Accountability and privacy protection
China	National Health Commission (NHC), PIPL (Personal Information Protection Law)	• AI product approval and clinical validation • PIPL for data protection	• Innovation and patient safety in healthcare AI • Comprehensive data protection standards and consent requirements
Japan	Ministry of Health, Labour, and Welfare (MHLW), PMDA (Pharmaceuticals and Medical Devices Agency)	• AI Health and Medical Strategy • Regulatory guidelines for AI-based medical devices	• Improving healthcare delivery through AI • Ethical standards for bias, transparency, and accountability in AI technologies
South Korea	Ministry of Food and Drug Safety (MFDS), PIPA (Personal Information Protection Act)	• AI-based medical device regulation • PIPA for data privacy	• Approval process for AI medical devices • Ensuring data security, patient consent, and algorithm transparency
Australia	Therapeutic Goods Administration (TGA), Privacy Act 1988	• SaMD guidelines • Privacy laws for health data	• Clinical validation and safety of AI devices • Transparent and reliable AI algorithms
New Zealand	MedSafe	• AI-based medical devices regulation • Ethical AI standards	• Safety and ethical deployment of AI devices • Bias prevention and data privacy

new data inputs. The FDA's current approach, such as its proposed Predetermined Change Control Plan for AI/ML-based Software as a Medical Device (SaMD) being developed together with Health Canada and the United Kingdom's Healthcare Products Regulatory Agency to serve as a set of guiding principles, attempts to address this by allowing predefined modifications without requiring new approvals for each change [25]. However, healthcare end users will still face the challenge of ensuring that updates and changes in AI models are safe, effective, and thoroughly tested, which may require ongoing regulatory oversight and continuous post-market monitoring. This could place a significant burden on healthcare providers who implement these products and developers of these systems to ensure compliance while keeping up with the pace of AI advancements.

Another challenge lies in addressing issues related to bias, transparency, and accountability in AI algorithms (see Chap. 10). AI systems are only as good as the data they are trained on, and biased data can lead to skewed outcomes that disproportionately affect certain populations, leading to ethical concerns. As the U.S. moves toward more comprehensive regulation, users can expect increasing requirements for transparency in how AI systems make decisions, as well as efforts to address and mitigate bias. However, ensuring transparency in complex AI systems, especially those that rely on deep learning algorithms, presents significant challenges since these systems often function as "black boxes" with decisions that are difficult to interpret. Users may also face regulatory expectations around accountability, where providers or developers could be held liable for decisions made by AI systems, particularly in cases where AI recommendations lead to adverse patient outcomes. Addressing these challenges in regulatory frameworks will require a delicate balance between fostering innovation and ensuring ethical, safe, and equitable use of AI in healthcare.

References

1. Palaniappan K, Lin EYT, Vogel S. Global regulatory frameworks for the use of artificial intelligence (AI) in the healthcare services sector. Healthcare (Basel). 2024;12(5):562.
2. U.S. Food and Drug Administration. Artificial Intelligence/Machine Learning (AI/ML)-Based Software as a Medical Device (SaMD) Action Plan. FDA; 2021. https://www.fda.gov/media/145022/download. Accessed 28 Sept 2024.
3. OpenRegulatory. FDA Risk Classification for Software as a Medical Device (SaMD). Published June 27, 2024. https://openregulatory.com/fda-risk-classification-for-software-as-a-medical-device-samd/. Accessed 29 Sept 2024.
4. U.S. Food and Drug Administration. Digital Health Software Precertification (Pre-Cert) Pilot Program. https://www.fda.gov/medical-devices/digital-health-center-excellence/digital-health-software-precertification-pre-cert-pilot-program. Accessed 29 Sept 2024.
5. U.S. Department of Health and Human Services. Health Insurance Portability and Accountability Act (HIPAA) Privacy Rule. https://www.hhs.gov/hipaa/for-professionals/privacy/index.html. Accessed 29 Sept 2024.

6. U.S. Department of Health and Human Services, Office for Civil Rights. Enforcement of the HIPAA Rules. Published July 26, 2013. https://www.hhs.gov/hipaa/for-professionals/compliance-enforcement/index.html. Accessed 29 Sept 2024.
7. International Organization for Standardization. ISO Standards. https://www.iso.org/standards.html. Accessed 29 Sept 2024.
8. Bello y Villarino J. Global standard-setting for artificial intelligence: para-regulating international law for AI? Aust Yearb Int Law Online. 2023;41(1):157–81.
9. American National Standards Institute (ANSI). ANSI overview. ANSI, the official U.S. representative to ISO. https://www.ansi.org. Accessed 29 Sept 2024.
10. ISO/IEC 23894:2023. Information Technology—Artificial Intelligence—Risk Management. AI Standards Hub. Published February 1, 2023. https://aistandardshub.org/ai-standards/information-technology-artificial-intelligence-risk-management/. Accessed 29 Sept 2024.
11. Meskó B, Topol EJ. The imperative for regulatory oversight of large language models (or generative AI) in healthcare. NPJ Digit Med. 2023;6:120.
12. Schmidt J, Schutte NM, Buttigieg S, Novillo-Ortiz D, Sutherland E, Anderson M, et al. Mapping the regulatory landscape for artificial intelligence in health within the European Union. NPJ Digit Med. 2024;7:229.
13. European Union. Regulation (EU) 2016/679 of the European Parliament and of the Council of 27 April 2016 on the protection of natural persons with regard to the processing of personal data and on the free movement of such data (General Data Protection Regulation). Off J Eur Union. 2016;L119:1–88.
14. European Union. Regulation (EU) 2017/745 of the European Parliament and of the Council of 5 April 2017 on medical devices, amending Directive 2001/83/EC, Regulation (EC) No 178/2002 and Regulation (EC) No 1223/2009, and repealing Council Directives 90/385/EEC and 93/42/EEC (Medical Device Regulation). Off J Eur Union. 2017;L117:1–175.
15. European Medicines Agency. Reflection paper on the use of Artificial Intelligence (AI) in the medicinal product lifecycle. Published July 13, 2023. https://www.ema.europa.eu/en/news/reflection-paper-use-artificial-intelligence-lifecycle-medicines. Accessed 29 Sept 2024.
16. Government of Canada. Personal Information Protection and Electronic Documents Act (S.C. 2000, c. 5). Updated June 20, 2024. https://laws-lois.justice.gc.ca/eng/acts/P-8.6/. Accessed 29 Sept 2024.
17. Health Canada. Pre-market guidance for machine learning-enabled medical devices. Published October 27, 2021. https://www.canada.ca/en/health-canada/services/drugs-health-products/medical-devices/application-information/guidance-documents/pre-market-guidance-machine-learning-enabled-medical-devices.html. Accessed 29 Sept 2024.
18. National Medical Products Administration (NMPA). Guiding principles for the classification and definition of AI-based medical software products. Published July 1, 2021. https://english.nmpa.gov.cn/2021-07/08/c_660267.htm. Accessed 29 Sept 2024.
19. Healthcare and medical devices 2024: trends and developments. Chambers Practice Guides. Published 2024. https://practiceguides.chambers.com/practice-guides/healthcare-medical-devices-2024/japan/trends-and-developments. Accessed 29 Sept 2024.
20. Ministry of Food and Drug Safety (MFDS). Guidance for the review and approval of artificial intelligence-based medical devices. Published September 2020. https://www.mfds.go.kr/eng/brd/m_40/view.do?seq=72627. Accessed 29 Sept 2024.
21. Therapeutic Goods Administration (TGA). Artificial Intelligence (AI) and Medical Device Software. Published February 25, 2021. https://www.tga.gov.au/how-we-regulate/manufacturing/manufacture-medical-device/manufacture-specific-types-medical-devices/artificial-intelligence-ai-and-medical-device-software. Accessed 29 Sept 2024.
22. Medsafe. Regulatory guidance for medical devices in New Zealand. Published October 23, 2019. https://www.medsafe.govt.nz/regulatory/DevicesNew/Industry.asp. Accessed 29 Sept 2024.

23. U.S. House of Representatives. Algorithmic Accountability Act of 2022, H.R. 6580, 117th Congress (2022). https://www.congress.gov/bill/117th-congress/house-bill/6580. Accessed 29 Sept 2024.
24. U.S. Senate. Advancing Artificial Intelligence Research Act of 2021, S. 3891, 116th Congress (2020). https://www.congress.gov/bill/116th-congress/senate-bill/3891/amendments. Accessed 29 Sept 2024.
25. U.S. Food and Drug Administration. Predetermined change control plans for machine learning-enabled medical devices: guiding principles. https://www.fda.gov/medical-devices/software-medical-device-samd/predetermined-change-control-plans-machine-learning-enabled-medical-devices-guiding-principles. Accessed 29 Sept 2024.

Part IV
Implementing Digital and AI Technologies in Medical Education and Clinical Settings

Chapter 15
Implementing Generative AI into Health Systems, Hospitals and Your Practice: Preparing for Change

Holly Urban

Introduction

While implementing any new technology in a healthcare setting is challenging, additional challenges may be encountered when implementing GenAI solutions. GenAI, while a powerful technology, is not a solution in and of itself. Healthcare organizations need a sound framework to evaluate whether the AI tool solves compelling clinical, operational, and/or financial challenges. Healthcare organizations also need to monitor performance of GenAI tools thoughtfully and deliberately, as these tools aren't "set it and forget it" solutions due to the risk of model drift, bias, and clinical validity.

In this chapter, a fictitious AI tool "NeoTPN" will serve as a case study to reinforce the concepts reviewed. "NeoTPN" is a GenAI tool that calculates lipids, proteins, carbohydrates, and micronutrients for pediatric and neonatal total parenteral nutrition (TPN) based on diagnoses, age, weight, and laboratory values.

Governance

While many healthcare systems are prioritizing investment in AI tools, 75% report insufficient planning or resources available to support their use [1]. GenAI tools hold the potential to move rapidly from niche technology solutions into widespread use with resultant behavioral and cultural changes [2]. Thus governance is foundational to ensure that these tools are selected, trialed, implemented, and monitored safely and ethically. Strong governance ensures patient safety and accountability by

H. Urban (✉)
Wolters Kluwer Health, Waltham, MA, USA
e-mail: Holly.Urban@wolterskluwer.com

T. Adirim (ed.), *Digital Health, AI and Generative AI in Healthcare*,
https://doi.org/10.1007/978-3-031-83526-1_15

the health system, as well as fostering clinician trust to improve adoption and achieve desired improvement in outcomes [3].

With decreasing budgets for all digital solutions, including AI tools, healthcare organizations need to have a comprehensive strategy to assess any new digital solution and a prioritization methodology. A few healthcare organizations have implemented a multidisciplinary oversight committee to thoroughly evaluate any proposed AI solution prior to its purchase or implementation. Governance bodies need to address the entire lifecycle of AI tools, including formal methods to evaluate potential solutions, implement, and perform continuous clinical validation [4]. The governance model should align with principles of risk stratification and quality management as described by the FDA [5]. See Chap. 14 for regulatory frameworks.

At Duke University, all algorithmic and AI tools must be registered with the Algorithm-Based Clinical Decision Support (ABCDS) Oversight multidisciplinary committee, which consists of clinical and operational leadership, biostatisticians, AI engineers, data scientists, as well as experts in law, regulation, and health equity. The oversight committee reviews all registrations and determines whether the tool can proceed to implementation and through a phase-gate process, discussed further below [6].

Assessing AI Solutions for Clinical Use

A broad range of commercial and non-commercial entities have brought a diverse landscape of AI solutions to the market. When evaluating new tools, it is recommended to adhere to the characteristics of trustworthy AI, as defined by NIST: valid and reliable, safe, secure and resilient, accountable and transparent, explainable and interpretable, privacy-enhanced, and fair with harmful bias managed [7].

Healthcare organizations should assess potential solutions against multiple dimensions, with clear attention to known issues such as safety and equity. The following are questions regarding evidence of effectiveness, appropriate uses, risk, vendor experience, and costs that institutions should answer prior to acquiring and implementing AI powered tools.

Evidence

Has evidence supporting the use of the tool been published in a peer-reviewed journal? Has the tool itself been evaluated in a randomized, controlled trial and shown a statistically significant benefit in clinical, operational, or financial outcomes? Many of the published studies evaluating AI tools involve observational studies which are not reproducible or biased in study design and methodology [8].

Use Case

Is the tool a solution looking for a problem, or does it address a well-understood, pervasive, compelling problem for the healthcare organization? What clinical, financial, or operational outcomes does the solution intend to achieve? What is the proposed workflow and user interface for the tool? How does it compare to the current state? What performance metrics can be used to monitor ongoing tool performance following implementation?

Risk

What is the potential risk to patient safety or harm related to use of the tool? What are the implications if the tool has an error or mistake in output? For GenAI applications that provide diagnostic support, such as providing differential diagnoses based on patient factors, what is the sensitivity or specificity of the tool? Highly sensitive tools will capture the majority of pertinent diagnoses but may lead to overdiagnosis (false positives) and "padding" of the list of differential diagnoses, impacting the clinical value. Whereas highly specific tools will capture accurate diagnoses but may miss diagnoses (false negatives), which increases the risk of omission.

Company and References

Is the vendor well established, with existing products in the market? Does the vendor have other customers using the AI tool? What was their experience, and do they have reference clients willing to directly discuss their experiences using the tool?

Cost

What are the costs of the solution, both from a licensing standpoint, as well as training and implementation costs? Will there be high costs related to ongoing support, especially considering the need for ongoing tool monitoring (discussed further below)? Does the anticipated improvement in outcomes justify the expense? While experts have advocated that reimbursement for AI services will be required to scale and financially sustain adoption of clinical AI, at the time of this writing, commercial or federal billing models for medical AI do not exist [9].

Regulatory Compliance

Does the tool require FDA clearance as Software as a Medical Device (SaMD)? Is IRB application required? Are data sharing agreements with the vendor required?

Technical Feasibility

What are the technical requirements and timelines? Where are the integration points? What is the anticipated data flow represented as a data flow diagram? What are plans for testing and evaluation of the tool?

Equity

What are potential sources of bias? What strategies are in place to prevent bias or mitigate harms from bias? What is the plan for ongoing monitoring and equity subgroup analysis?

Alignment with Long-Term Strategy

Organizational motivation, described as the how the tool aligns with organizational goals, resources, and support, has been shown to be a strong predictor of successful implementations [10]. Healthcare organizations moving toward value-based care need to be aware that the landscape of AI and digital solutions primarily focus on disease treatment, mirroring US healthcare fee-for-service reimbursement models. A cross-sectional study of US based digital health solutions showed that nearly three-quarters of digital health companies focused on management of disease, while the minority addressed prevention or detection of disease [11]. Any potential digital tool should preferably support disease prevention or population health if the goal of the healthcare organization is to move to value-based care contracts.

Healthcare organizations may find it useful to use a standard framework to assess digital health tools. The evaluation framework provides a semi-quantitative method to standardize the evaluation of digital health tools across different dimensions and allow prioritization when multiple tools are under consideration (see Table 15.1). Tools are weighted against each category with higher scores indicating higher desirability of the tool for the health system.

Table 15.1 Sample evaluation framework

Category	Ambient listening (EHR vendor)	Fax summaries (XYZ company)	TPN orders (NeoTPN)
Evidence Rating	3	1	3
Use Case	5	3	1
Risk	5	5	1
Company Status	5	3	1
Cost	1	3	5
Regulatory Oversight	5	5	3
Technical Feasibility	5	3	1
Equity	3	3	1
Strategy	3	3	3
Total	35	29	19

Key:
Evidence rating—5 = multiple randomized controlled trials, 3 = one randomized controlled trial or multiple observational trials, 1 = one observational trial
Use case—5 = Addresses a significant problem for most clinical users, 3 = Addresses a significant problem for some clinical users, 1 = Addresses a significant problem for few clinical users
Risk—5 = low to no risk, 3 = medium risk, 1 = high risk
Company Status—5 = Well established company with multiple users of solution, 3 = Well established company with few pilot users or new company with multiple users, 1 = New/start-up company with few pilot users
Cost—5 = Low cost to license, implement, and maintain, 3 = medium cost to license, implement, and maintain, 1 = high cost to license, implement, and maintain
Regulatory Oversight—5 = no regulatory oversight, 3 = IRB oversight, 1 = FDA oversight
Technical Feasibility—5 = low to no resources or technical effort required, 3 = medium resources or technical effort required, 1 = high resources or technical effort required
Equity—5 = no risks or harms from bias, 3 = medium or unknown risk from bias, 1 = high risk from bias
Strategy – 5 = highly aligned with organization's long-term strategy, 3 = somewhat aligned with strategy, 1 = not aligned with strategy.
Note: Own work

Implementation Strategies

The meaningful impact of digital innovations, such as GenAI tools, relies not only on the effectiveness of the tool, but also on its proper implementation, distribution, and broad spread adoption [12]. Implementation science provides a framework to translate research and new tools into routine practice and practical outcomes [13]. As noted in Fig. 15.1, successful implementation of a tool into broad clinical practice and culture requires multiple phases.

The complexity of AI tools in terms of clinician acceptance, workflow impact, ongoing monitoring, and patient safety, requires a higher bar for implementation than more straightforward implementation of medical devices or other digital tools. The SAFER Guides, published by the Office of the National Coordinator for Health

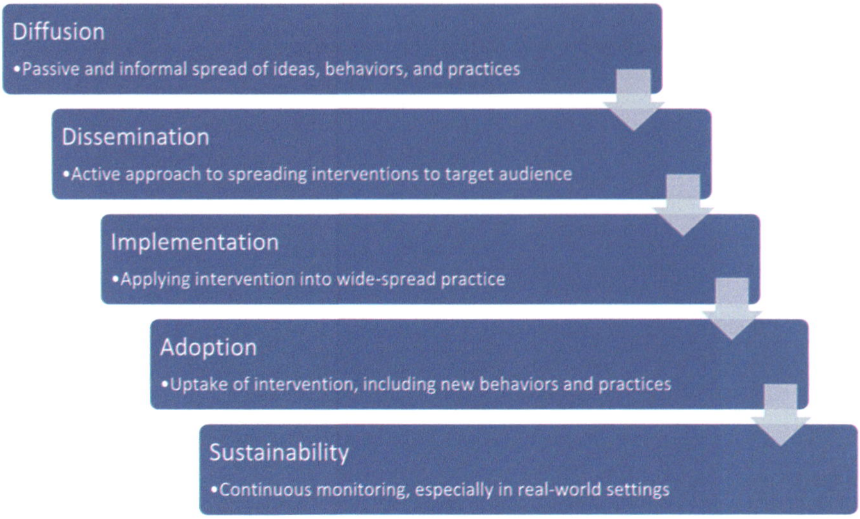

Fig. 15.1 Phases of implementation. *Adapted from Rapport, 2018* [13]

Information Technology to enable implementation of Electronic Health Records (EHR), can be utilized to focus on patient safety when implementing AI tools [14]. The SAFER Guides allow organizations to do self-assessment in nine areas to evaluate the safe use of EHRs, such as High Priority Practices and Organizational Responsibilities, that can be leveraged for evaluation of AI tool readiness.

The Veteran's Administration published a practical playbook for implementation in real-world settings, "Getting to Implementation (GTI)." The GTI playbook includes, in addition to introductory materials supporting the intervention for healthcare organization leadership, materials to support a stepwise approach to implementation: [15].

- Build a dedicated team and identify current practices, including process mapping of current state clinical workflows compared to future state workflows.
- Establish goals and evidence-based practice of the intervention.
- Assess strengths and barriers and prioritize barriers using a Barriers Prioritization Tool.
- Choose best-practice solutions and strategies for implementation.
- Plan and adapt solutions, including assessing readiness to implement.
- Implement, evaluate, and improve based on monitoring of pre-determined metrics.
- Sustain, review, and look ahead.

Duke University created implementation guides to facilitate implementation of AI models with oversight from the ABCDS Oversight Governance Committee, as described above. The implementation guide describes a phased gate process whereby the AI tool is evaluated at multiple checkpoints [6]:

- G0 checkpoint after model development: Initial registration, with initial criteria evaluating transparency and accountability, clinical value and safety, fairness and equity, usability and adoption, and regulatory compliance.
- G1 checkpoint after silent evaluation period: Registration updates following a silent evaluation period with real time patient data ensuring technical data flow, algorithm performance, and plan for a limited pilot deployment (effectiveness evaluation) that includes workflow diagrams and end user evaluation.
- G2 checkpoint after effectiveness evaluation: Updates that critically assess the small-scale pilot, with plans for maintenance and ongoing monitoring that include metrics for clinical impact and equity.
- Gm checkpoint during general deployment: Periodic check ins and continuous algorithm monitoring following general deployment of the tool.

Training

The KLAS Arch Collaborative, a consortium of over 250 healthcare organizations focused on EHR optimization, studied the reasons clinician satisfaction varied greatly between health systems using the same Electronic Health Record and found that inadequate training was one of the largest drivers of poor satisfaction [16]. Training can help provider adoption of tools through not only competency and proficiency of tool use, but also facilitate building trust between providers and patients [17].

However, plans for training need to reflect the overall impact to established workflows, especially if the new tool impacts team-based care processes. When the new tool involves hand offs in care, individual training is insufficient, as process workflow design and training on new processes are required. With new processes, staffing may also need to change. Thus, any new tool impacting team-based care processes needs team-based training, so everyone understands the hand offs and the implications of hand offs.

For example, when implementing an AI tool that triages patient portal communication to nurses instead of all patient messages going directly to provider inboxes, the organization should clearly depict the workflow with message entry points, the criteria for routing messages, and the staffing pool to handle routed messages, all of which need to be incorporated into team-based training. This approach will allow physicians and nurses to be comfortable with the triage, workflow, and how hand offs are managed.

Supportive Resources

The presence of "super users" or "physician champions" during the early phases of implementation have proven to improve adoption of new tools. A clinician led approach can mitigate resistance [18]. When selecting resources to serve in these roles, they should be influential staff level individuals with extensive social capital to invest in engendering adoption, not low producers who might not be "missed" if their clinical time is reduced while performing in a super user role.

Individuals who have both contextual understanding of local workflows and who are well trained on the new technology improve mediation of adoption and use, suggesting healthcare organizations invest in training on the technology and explicit programs to develop mediation skills of their employees to aid implementation and adoption [19].

Change Management

The hype associated with GenAI may render a negative impression and create a barrier to adoption for clinical end users. Popular media frequently publishes stories about hallucinations, causing generalized mistrust of GenAI technology. Physicians struggle with the potential impact of AI on patient-physician relationships and "the professional integrity of physicians." [20] Many physicians have concerns about liability when an AI model provides misleading or wrong information. In May 2024, The Federation of State Medical Boards adopted policy that states that physicians are "responsible for the use of AI and should be held accountable for any harms that occur." [21].

Physicians may fear that any improvements in productivity gained as a result of GenAI efficiency tools may translate into management expectations for a greater patient load. Finally, physicians, nurses and other providers may fear that AI models will effectively replace them. Geoffrey Hinton, a deep learning pioneer, stated at an AI conference that within 5 years deep learning would replace radiologists [22]. Regarding these concerns, change management needs to not only address fear of change, but fear of the technology itself.

Concrete strategies to advance change management with physicians and other clinicians:

- *Getting to Why* Healthcare organizations should clearly communicate to physicians the stated clinical or efficiency outcomes to be achieved as a result of the AI tool. Physicians pursue a challenging path to become a physician and are motivated to provide great patient care. The same for others responsible for healthcare delivery such as nurses. They are also interested in how they can become more efficient in their daily tasks, reducing burnout, and freeing time to focus on patients. Tying the improved clinical or efficiency outcomes tied to the GenAI tool helps reinforce those altruistic goals. Citing financial or operational outcomes may be less compelling to clinician end users.
- *Provide Data* Physicians are trained in the scientific method and respond well to data-driven rationale for deploying a given AI tool. For example, when NYU Langone embarked on an AI data-driven quality improvement initiative to

improve clinical notes, leadership justified the necessity for improvement by sharing data with physicians about the high prevalence of poor-quality notes [23].

- *Identify Champions* As discussed above, identifying people who are well trained in the technology and understand the local workflow can successfully aid adoption [19]. Having a fellow, trusted physician as a vocal advocate of the tool who can socialize its benefits leads to increased trust and improved adoption among his/her peers.
- *Reassurance* Leadership needs to communicate that using AI tools will not lead to higher patient volumes or physician layoffs, and that the intention of AI tools is to improve quality of care and patient outcomes.

Case Study: NeoTPN

- Prior to initiating training, hospital leadership informed the physician staff that NeoTPN was studied in a randomized, controlled trial that showed neonates and children on NeoTPN had statistically lower incidences of hyperglycemia, hyperlipidemia, and elevated liver function tests than the control group managed by traditional methods.
- A recent audit indicated that in their facility, 15% of TPN orders were incorrectly ordered and 2% of TPN orders were associated with an adverse outcome.
- One of the neonatologists at the facility led the trial which showed improved outcomes, and vocally supported its use among other neonatologists, neonatal nurse practitioners, pharmacists, and dieticians, which improved adoption.
- Leadership supported the use of NeoTPN, endorsing the improved outcomes for a vulnerable patient population.

Formal assessment of readiness for change can be accomplished using surveys initiated prior to implementation. Organizational change theory suggests that assessing readiness for change can facilitate successful adoption, which requires changes in the workflows of staff and often realignment of roles [24]. Two instruments, Normalization MeAsure Development questionnaire (NoMAD) [25] and Organizational Readiness for Implementing Change (ORIC) [26], both reliably predicted the success of implementing interventions into practice [27]. These instruments can be adapted for relevancy of the specific AI tool being implemented.

Monitoring AI Tools

Healthcare organizations need robust methods for the ongoing evaluation and monitoring of the performance of AI Tools. There are critical reasons for ongoing monitoring:

- *Model Overfitting* Overfitting occurs when the AI model "learned" on a training development sample that is not generalizable to other settings [28]. AI Models trained on a limited, discrete data set during their development may not translate well to a different healthcare setting, time, or population.
- *Hallucinations* The tendency for GenAI tools to manufacture content serves as one of the most challenging aspects in healthcare applications of GenAI, when certainty and precision of information is paramount. Current techniques such as Retrieval Augmented Generation (RAG) [29] specifically restrict source data to improve the accuracy and fidelity of the information generated. For many healthcare applications of GenAI, end users can flag or otherwise mark 'incorrect' outputs. These flags should be monitored zealously by the organization so if significant errors occur, the tool developers can address the issue and/or the tool can be removed from clinical usage.
- *Equity* Concern regarding perpetuating bias in healthcare Gen AI applications may limit acceptability of its recommendations in clinical practice. Four domains to consider include sex, race/ethnicity, age, and insurance status. Issues with unequal access for under-resourced sites of care can be addressed using a metric such as "population achieved sensitivity." [30] Bias auditing tools leverage multiple methods to mitigate bias, such as fairness metrics, counterfactual analysis, sensitivity analysis across demographic subgroups, algorithmic transparency, and adversarial testing [31]. Any technical solution to reduce bias will have its own limitations and ultimately the best method may be in human diligence in searching for bias [32].
- *Outcomes* Performance metrics should be selected prior to implementation, and ideally monitored pre- and post-implementation. Ongoing monitoring for the desired clinical, operational, or financial outcomes of GenAI tools will help determine ROI. Outcomes should be communicated broadly to AI Governance bodies, healthcare organization leadership, and to end users. Understanding the concrete outcomes of AI models can also establish the groundwork for go-forward application of related GenAI tools.

Ongoing safety assessment is paramount, as the nature of GenAI tools allows them to learn and adapt over time, meaning that after testing and initial evaluation, different results could result from the tool after implementation and ongoing use [33]. Embi (2021) described an ethical imperative for healthcare systems to perform "algorithmovigilance," invoking the "methods and activities relating to the evaluation, monitoring, understanding, and prevention of adverse effects of algorithms in health care." [34].

Conclusion

As with any digital tool, implementing medical AI tools must involve the careful selection of tools that clearly demonstrate improvements to clinical, financial, or operational outcomes. Due to the inherent risks of medical AI tools with model drift, hallucinations, and bias, careful implementation and ongoing monitoring of tool performance is critical. Governance and oversight of these tools serve to protect the health system from inherent risks as well as to gain clinician buy-in. Clear communication, training, and leveraging best practice change management approaches will allow niche technology solutions to achieve the cultural and clinical benefits hoped for with medical AI.

References

1. Eastburn J, Fowkes J, Kellner K, Swanson B. Digital transformation: health systems' investment priorities. McKinsey & Company. 2024. https://www.mckinsey.com/industries/healthcare/our-insights/digital-transformation-health-systems-investmentpriorities. Accessed 14 June 2024.
2. Durlach P, Fournier R, Gottlich J, Markwell T, McManus J, Merrill A, et al. The AI maturity roadmap: a framework for effective and sustainable AI in health care. NEJM AI. 2024; https://ai.nejm.org/doi/full/10.1056/AI-S2400177. Accessed June 6, 2024
3. Liao F, Adelaine S, Afshar M, Patterson B. Governance of Clinical AI applications to facilitate safe and equitable deployment in a large health system: key elements and early successes. Front Digit Health. 2022;8:931439.
4. Bedoya AD, Economou-Zavlanos NJ, Goldstein BA, Young A, Jelovsek JE, O'Brien C, et al. A framework for the oversight and local deployment of safe and high-quality prediction models. J Am Med Inform Assoc. 2022;29(9):1631–6.
5. US Food and Drug Administration (FDA). Artificial Intelligence and Machine Learning in software as a medical device. https://www.fda.gov/medical-devices/software-medical-device-samd/artificial-intelligence-and-machine-learning-software-medical-device. Accessed 3 June 2024.
6. Economou-Zavlanos NJ, Bessias S, Cary MP Jr, Bedoya AD, Goldstein BA, Jelovsek JE, et al. Translating ethical and quality principles for the effective, safe, and fair development, deployment, and use of artificial intelligence technologies in healthcare. J Am Med Inform Assoc. 2024;31(3):705–13.
7. National Institutes of Standards and Technology (NIST). Artificial Intelligence Risk Management Framework (AI RMF 1.0). 2023. https://nvlpubs.nist.gov/nistpubs/ai/NIST.AI.100-1.pdf. Accessed 10 June 2024.
8. Byrne DW, Domenico HJ, Moore RP. Artificial intelligence for improved patient outcomes-the pragmatic randomized controlled trial is the secret sauce. Korean J Radiol. 2024;25(2):123–5.
9. Abramoff MD, Dai T, Zou J. Scaling adoption of medical AI—reimbursement from value-based care and fee-for-service perspectives. NEJM AI. 2024;1(5). https://doi.org/10.1056/AIpc2400083.
10. Wen K, Gustafson DH, Hawkin RP, Brennan PF, Dinauer S, Johnson PR, et al. Developing and validating a model to predict the success of an IHCS implementation: the Readiness for Implementation Model. J Am Med Inform Assoc. 2010;17(6):707–13.
11. Cohen AB, Dorsey ER, Mathews SC, Bates DW, Safavi K. A digital health industry cohort across the health continuum. NPJ Digit Med. 2020;3(68). https://doi.org/10.1038/s41746-020-0276-9.
12. Fernandez ME, Ten Hoor GA, van Lieshout S, Rodriguez SA, Beidas RS, Parcel G, et al. Implementation mapping: using intervention mapping to develop implementation strategies. Front Public Health. 2019;7(158):158.
13. Rapport F, Clay-Williams R, Churruca K, Shih P, Hogden A, Braithwaite J. The struggle of translating science into action: foundational concepts of implementation science. J Eval Clin Pract. 2018;24(1):117–26.

14. Office of the National Coordinator for Health Information Technology (ONC). SAFER Guides. https://www.healthit.gov/topic/safety/safer-guides. Accessed 3 June 2024.
15. Yakovchenko V, Rogal SS, Goodrich DE, Lamorte C, Neely B, Merante M, et al. Getting to implementation: adaptation of an implementation playbook. Front Public Health. 2023;10:980958.
16. KLAS Arch Collaborative. https://klasresearch.com/arch-collaborative. Accessed 10 June 2024.
17. Ramachandran M, Brinton C, Wiljer D, Upshur R, Gray CS. The impact of eHealth on relationships and trust in primary care: a review of reviews. BMC Prim Care. 2023;24(228). https://doi.org/10.1186/s12875-023-02176-5.
18. Banas CA, Erskine AR, Sun S, Retchin SM. Phased implementation of electronic health records through an office of clinical transformation. J Am Med Inform Assoc. 2011;18(5):721–5.
19. Umstead CN, Unertl KM, Lorenzi NM, Novak LL. Enabling adoption and use of new health information technology during implementation: roles and strategies for internal and external support personnel. J Am Med Inform Assoc. 2021;28(7):1543–7.
20. Daneshvar N, Pandita D, Erickson S, Sulmasy LS, DeCamp M. ACP Medical Informatics Committee and the Ethics, Professionalism and Human Rights Committee. Artificial Intelligence in the Provision of Health Care: An American College of Physicians Policy Position Paper. Ann Intern Med. 2024;177(7):964–7.
21. Federation of State Medical Boards. Navigating the responsible and ethical incorporation of Artificial Intelligence into clinical practice. https://www.fsmb.org/siteassets/advocacy/policies/incorporation-of-ai-into-practice.pdf. Accessed 3 June 2024.
22. Hinton G. Geoff Hinton: on radiology. https://www.youtube.com/watch?v=2HMPRXstSvQ. November 24, 2016. Accessed 3 June 2024.
23. Feldman J, Hockman K, Guzman BV, Goodman A, Weisstuch J, Testa P. Scaling note quality assessment across an academic medical center with AI and GPT-4. NEJM Catal Innov Care Deliv. 2024;5(5). https://doi.org/10.1056/CAT.23.0283.
24. Wen K, Gustafson DH, Hawkins RP, Brennan PF, Dinauer S, Johnson PR, et al. Developing and validating a model to predict the success of an IHCS implementation: the Readiness for Implementation Model. J Am Med Inform Assoc. 2010;17(6):707–13.
25. Finch TL, Girling M, May CR, et al. NoMAD: Implementation measure based on Normalization Process Theory. [Measurement instrument]. 2015. http://www.normalizationprocess.org. Accessed 14 June 2024.
26. Shea CM, Jacobs SR, Esserman DA, Bruce K, Weiner BJ. Organizational Readiness for implementing change: a psychometric assessment of a new measure. Implement Sci. 2014;20(7). https://doi.org/10.1186/1748-5908-9-7. https://www.implementall.eu/ORIC_English.pdf. Accessed 14 June 2024.
27. Batterham P, Allenhof C, Cerga Pashoj A, Etzelmueller A, Fanaj N, Finch T, et al. Psychometric properties of two implementation measures: normalization MeAsure Development questionnaire (NoMAD) and organizational readiness for implementing change (ORIC). Implement Res Pract. 2024;5. https://doi.org/10.1177/26334895241245448.
28. Mutasa S, Sun S, Ha R. Understanding artificial intelligence-based radiology studies: what is overfitting? Clin Imaging. 2020;65:96–9.
29. Miao J, Thongprayoon C, Suppadungsuk S, Garcia Valencia OA, Cheungpasitporn W. Integrating retrieval-augmented generation with large language models in nephrology: advancing practical applications. Medicina (Kaunas). 2024;60(3):445.
30. Abràmoff MD, Tarver ME, Loyo-Berrios N, Trujillo S, Char D, Obermeyer Z, et al. Considerations for addressing bias in artificial intelligence for health equity. NPJ Digit Med. 2023;6:170.
31. Chen Y, Clayton EW, Novak LL, Anders S, Malin B. Human-centered design to address biases in artificial intelligence. J Med Internet Res. 2023;25:e43251.

32. Franklin G, Stephens R, Piracha M, Tiosano S, Lehouillier F, Koppel R, et al. The sociodemographic biases in machine learning algorithms: a biomedical informatics perspective. Life. 2024;14(6):652.
33. Adams L, Fontaine E, Lin S, Crowell T, Chung VCH, Gonzalez AA, editors. 2024. Artificial intelligence in health, health care and biomedical science: An AI code of conduct framework principles and commitments discussion draft. NAM Perspectives. Commentary, National Academy of Medicine, Washington, DC. https://doi.org/10.31478/202403a.
34. Embi PJ. Algorithmovigilance—advancing methods to analyze and monitor artificial intelligence–driven health care for effectiveness and equity. JAMA Netw Open. 2021;4(4):e214622.

Chapter 16
Digital Technology for Medical Education

Taylor Freeburg and Todd P. Chang

Introduction

In recent years, the field of medical education has undergone a profound transformation, primarily driven by advancements in digital technology. The social distancing limitations due to the COVID-19 pandemic catalyzed unprecedented developments in digital technologies and have revolutionized how students learn, practitioners stay current, and healthcare systems deliver care.

Digital technology encompasses an array of tools and platforms, ranging from podcasts to serious games and virtual anatomy applications (apps). These technologies offer unprecedented opportunities for experiential learning and skill development. Moreover, they facilitate personalized learning pathways, allowing students to engage with content at their own pace and according to their learning styles. Educators can harness digital tools to create immersive and interactive learning experiences, bridging the gap between theory and practice.

However, integrating digital technology into medical education is not without challenges. Issues such as digital literacy among faculty and students, the validity of content, and the potential for information overload require careful consideration and proactive management.

This chapter starts by exploring the integration of digital tools for student use, including podcasts, serious games, and anatomy applications. The chapter then addresses the role of artificial intelligence within medical education for trainees and clinical educators alike.

T. Freeburg (✉)
Department of Pediatrics, Children's Hospital Los Angeles, Los Angeles, CA, USA
e-mail: tfreeburg@chla.usc.edu

T. P. Chang
Department of Pediatrics, Division of Emergency Medicine & Transport,
Keck School of Medicine of USC, Los Angeles, CA, USA

T. Adirim (ed.), *Digital Health, AI and Generative AI in Healthcare*,
https://doi.org/10.1007/978-3-031-83526-1_16

Digital Technologies in Medical Education

Student/Trainee Uses for Digital Tech in Med Ed

Although digital technology has been present in medical education for years, it became universally used for preclinical education during the COVID-19 pandemic as medical schools used digital modalities to meet the demands of online learning. Digital technologies make medical education more accessible, standardized, relevant, timely, and affordable. Digital technologies potentially save resources for instructors by reducing facility costs (as students can complete the coursework remotely) and when using free or low-cost digital applications for learning [1]. Beyond a student's home medical school-curated content, students independently seek digital resources developed by other institutions during their clinical rotations [2]. Instructors could optimize learning using multiple digital technology modalities outlined below when building a curriculum.

Modalities and Media

Online Webpage Web-based online resources remain a staple for medical education, with various website content, including online textbooks, online calculators, and clinical decision-making cognitive aids. These tend to be very easily accessible and easily updated. Because of their static nature, interactivity, and the ability to explain complex topics may be challenging.

Webcasts e-learning modalities can be synchronous or asynchronous, typically with an expert's slide-based presentation (e.g., Microsoft PowerPoint). Webcasts allow for on-demand access to information. Strengths include the ability to view lectures more than once and the ability to restart, rewind, and pause lectures. Disadvantages include a lack of opportunity to ask questions if they are not synchronous and being subject to distractions. Vaccani et al. found improved written exam scores among medical students using this modality [3]. Similarly, knowledge scores improved with specified e-learning modules in a multi-center pediatric emergency department rotation among residents [4].

Video Video-based education enables certain complex concepts to be better explained and is another asynchronous medium for medical education. YouTube is an online website that allows users to view, upload, and share originally created videos. It is a medium that can provide up-to-date information as opposed to textbooks that on average, can take 1–3 years to publish. However, the downside of videos on YouTube is that they lack *peer* review. One study analyzed the content on human heart anatomy on YouTube and found only 25% of videos passed their preset level of accuracy [5]. More peer review and methods of vouching accuracy are necessary to include YouTube videos in medical education course content.

Anatomy Applications Many studies evaluating the feasibility and effectiveness of digital anatomy education applications are present in medical education literature [6, 7]. Technology has a wide variety of uses in augmenting or replacing cadaveric anatomical education. Anatomy curricula are creating blended learning environments, combining the cadaver learning experience with online activities. For example, online lecture webcasts using a teaching assistant can manipulate 3D computer models in a virtual classroom environment. Attardi et al. describe how students value pace control, schedule, and location flexibility of learning from online material but ultimately prefer hands-on experience with cadaveric specimens [8]. Therefore, digital, and virtual reality tools can be adjuncts but are not ideal substitutes for learning anatomy [9, 10].

Digital solutions for anatomy education include life-size virtual dissection tablets using 3D digital models of human cadaveric images and digital anatomy applications usable on devices outside the cadaver laboratory. Some examples of applications (apps) include Visible Body, 3D4Medical, and Pocket Anatomy [7, 11]. Advantages of digital anatomy apps include selective revealing of systems and regions of the body with the ability to reverse dissection. Details can be built, including labeling the origin, insertion, innervation, and vascular supply of muscles. Educators can use these apps by sharing the screen of their tablet on a projector to supplement cadaver dissections [11]. Digital anatomy instruction can substantially increase the available number of learners by using screen casting that can allow for massive open online courses (MOOCs) [12, 13]. However, technologies have not replicated the tactile haptics a human cadaver can provide. Among medical students, there are mixed preferences on the hands-on nature of learning on cadavers as opposed to a preference for the digital version of learning anatomy [8, 14].

Audio Podcast While video instruction enables complex ideas to be played out visually, audio instruction has enabled a different paradigm of education, in which education can occur in shorter periods of time and outside of the classroom, often while engaged in other activities such as while in transit and doing chores, to maximize time efficiency. Podcasts are playing an increasing role in medical education for medical students and residents and have become integrated into formal curricula. Podcasts are available in almost every specialty and have a widespread impact [15]. For example, the internal medicine podcast The Curbsiders, which uses expert interviews to discuss practice-changing knowledge for internists, averages over 40,000 downloads per episode [16]. Podcast producers include not only individual practitioners and educators (e.g., The Curbsiders, Annals on Call, Core IM, Bedside Rounds, Clinical Problem Solvers) but also influential medical journals (e.g., JAMA, NEJM, Annals of Internal Medicine). A scoping review found significant gaps in research about their optimal use and effectiveness. The review found that the strengths included that these podcasts were flexible, provided self-defined learning, and were entertaining [17]. The review suggests that advanced learners find podcasts more valuable than medical students, and podcasts have become common vehicles for Continuing Medical Education (CME) and Maintenance of Certification (MOC) credits for practicing physicians [16].

Serious Games and Gamification Serious Games are the use of a game not for entertainment but for teaching or simulating a concept. This contrasts with gamification, which uses game elements to increase engagement and facilitate learning. Games and gamification have been shown to positively impact student engagement, learning, and retention of knowledge [18, 19]. Examples of serious games include screen-based computer games or Virtual Reality-based simulations [20–22].

Gamification elements have become more popular with a variety of new software to increase engagement: PollEverywhere (PollEverywhere, United States), functions as an add-in software for MS PowerPoint, Apple Keynote, or Google Slides, which allows participants to respond to questions. Learner polling software has been used by different subspecialty fellowship training programs and resulted in more favorable satisfaction scores and self-perceived attentiveness [23]. One study using Kahoot! (Kahoot!, Norway), a trivia game-based learning platform to create and play learning games or quizzes, showed improved collaborative learning, knowledge of content, attendance, and participation. However, the researchers found negative outcomes for users including being overwhelmed by content learning content, and distractions due to gadgets [24].

Implementing New Digital Education Tools for Education

Technology is no longer only being used as a teaching tool but has become a crucial component of curricular development. The successful integration of digital technologies depends on the instructor's ability to merge new technologies with previous teaching modalities and the flexibility to change the curriculum as new digital technologies emerge. Barriers to incorporating digital technologies include the rapid evolution of technologies, limited funding, and varying levels of institutional support. One way to overcome these challenges is to involve student input when developing a curriculum. Shenson et al. describe a novel medical-student-led and faculty-sponsored technology committee that led to rapid improvements in educational technologies that met students' needs and enhanced learning opportunities [25].

Artificial Intelligence in Medical Education

Artificial intelligence (AI) has the potential to revolutionize medical education for both trainees and practicing physicians by streamlining and simplifying previously time-consuming tasks. Potential applications include conducting research, writing letters of recommendation and evaluations, crafting virtual patient simulations or case studies, and developing intelligent learning plans. Below is a detailed but not exhaustive list of the ways that artificial intelligence can be applied within the scope of medical education.

Modalities

- *Letters of Recommendation.* Chatbots like ChatGPT (OpenAI) employ machine learning algorithms to generate text and have the potential to ease the burden of writing letters of recommendation for residency training and academic promotion. Users can input a candidate's achievements into a prompt and receive a cohesively written letter of recommendation in response. A study by Preiksaitis et al. found that academic physicians were not reliably able to distinguish between human and AI-generated letters of recommendation [26]. Since AI natural language processing has been used in literature to analyze recommendation letter content for bias, authors have suggested that AI can generate letters with reduced implicit bias compared to the human counterpart; however, contrary arguments and data exist [27–29]. A significant research gap remains regarding AI's effectiveness and role in such professional evaluations within academia. Training in how to write effective input and prompts may improve the quality of letters that AI can generate, as output quality is contingent on the quality of the input [30].
- *Classroom Education.* AI can be used in the classroom setting as an assistant to educators and tutor to students. Studies have challenged ChatGPT to answer biomedical and clinical questions (in both multiple-choice and open-ended formats) derived from the United States Medical Licensing Examination and found that ChatGPT performed at or near passing with a high level of insight in its explanations to open-ended questions, suggesting that large language models have the potential to support students in the medical education field [31, 32]. Multiple studies have described how ChatGPT can be used to develop clinical vignettes with varying levels of complexity and can be directed to include specific case content to align with learning objectives [33, 34]. AI can also generate summaries, quizzes, and flashcards to facilitate learning and can be used as a virtual tutor to provide student feedback [35].
- *Research.* Within research, AI is a promising tool for both academic writing and the research process. ChatGPT can assist with formulating the research problem, reviewing relevant literature, selecting an appropriate research design, and collecting, analyzing, and interpreting data [36]. Regarding the academic writing process, studies have shown the potential for AI to propose outlines and generate early drafts of scientific publications [37–39].

Ethics of AI in Medical Education

There are many opportunities to integrate AI into medical education to reduce the burden of time-consuming tasks. Ethically, institutions will need to determine whether to disclose the use of AI within medical education [40, 41]. Busch et al. explore the biomedical ethical responsibilities to consider when implementing AI into medical education, including the importance of providing appropriate training, including offline and online workshops, for educators and students to understand how and when to use each application [42].

Conclusion

The integration of digital technologies in medical education has significantly transformed the learning experience. Educators can create more engaging and effective learning environments by embracing innovative tools such as podcasts, serious games, virtual anatomy applications, webcasts, and videos. The future potential for artificial intelligence in medical education holds promise for further advancements. However, challenges such as digital literacy, content validity, and potential information overload need to be carefully addressed. Looking ahead, the future of digital technology in medical education holds promise and excitement. Ultimately, as digital technology continues to evolve, its role in medical education will expand, shaping the future of healthcare delivery and professional development.

References

1. Sormunen M, Saaranen T, Heikkilä A, Sjögren T, Koskinen C, Mikkonen K, et al. Digital learning interventions in higher education: a scoping review. Comput Inform Nurs. 2020;38(12):613–24.
2. Scott K, Morris A, Marais B. Medical student use of digital learning resources. Clin Teach. 2018;15(1):29–33.
3. Vaccani JP, Javidnia H, Humphrey-Murto S. The effectiveness of webcast compared to live lectures as a teaching tool in medical school. Med Teach. 2016;38(1):59–63.
4. Chang TP, Pham PK, Sobolewski B, Doughty CB, Jamal N, Kwan KY, et al. Pediatric emergency medicine asynchronous e-learning: a multicenter randomized controlled Solomon four-group study. Acad Emerg Med. 2014;21(8):912–9.
5. Raikos A, Waidyasekara P. How useful is YouTube in learning heart anatomy? Anat Sci Educ. 2014;7(1):12–8.
6. Harmon DJ, Burgoon JM, Kalmar EL. Development and assessment of an integrated anatomy mobile app. Clin Anat. 2022;35(5):686–96.
7. Golenhofen N, Heindl F, Grab-Kroll C, Messerer DAC, Böckers TM, Böckers A. The use of a mobile learning tool by medical students in undergraduate anatomy and its effects on assessment outcomes. Anat Sci Educ. 2020;13(1):8–18.

8. Attardi SM, Choi S, Barnett J, Rogers KA. Mixed methods student evaluation of an online systemic human anatomy course with laboratory. Anat Sci Educ. 2016;9(3):272–85.
9. Ail G, Freer F, Chan CS, Jones M, Broad J, Canale GP, et al. A comparison of virtual reality anatomy models to prosections in station-based anatomy teaching. Anat Sci Educ. 2024;17(4):763–9.
10. Erolin C, Reid L, McDougall S. Using virtual reality to complement and enhance anatomy education. J Vis Commun Med. 2019;42(3):93–101.
11. Lewis TL, Burnett B, Tunstall RG, Abrahams PH. Complementing anatomy education using three-dimensional anatomy mobile software applications on tablet computers. Clin Anat. 2014;27(3):313–20.
12. Pickering JD, Swinnerton BJ. Exploring the dimensions of medical student engagement with technology-enhanced learning resources and assessing the impact on assessment outcomes. Anat Sci Educ. 2019;12(2):117–28.
13. Swinnerton BJ, Morris NP, Hotchkiss S, Pickering JD. The integration of an anatomy massive open online course (MOOC) into a medical anatomy curriculum. Anat Sci Educ. 2017;10(1):53–67.
14. Triepels CPR, Smeets CFA, Notten KJB, Kruitwagen RFPM, Futterer JJ, Vergeldt TFM, et al. Does three-dimensional anatomy improve student understanding? Clin Anat. 2020;33(1):25–33.
15. Little A, Hampton Z, Gronowski T, Meyer C, Kalnow A. Podcasting in medicine: a review of the current content by specialty. Cureus. 2020;12(1):e6726.
16. Berk J, Trivedi SP, Watto M, Williams P, Centor R. Medical education podcasts: where we are and questions unanswered. J Gen Intern Med. 2020;35(7):2176–8.
17. Kelly JM, Perseghin A, Dow AW, Trivedi SP, Rodman A, Berk J. Learning through listening: a scoping review of podcast use in medical education. Acad Med. 2022;97(7):1079–85.
18. Rutledge C, Walsh CM, Swinger N, Auerbach M, Castro D, Dewan M, et al. Gamification in action: theoretical and practical considerations for medical educators. Acad Med. 2018;93(7):1014–20.
19. Sailer M, Homner L. The gamification of learning: a meta-analysis. Educ Psychol Rev. 2020;32:77–112.
20. Luu C, Talbot TB, Fung CC, Ben-Isaac E, Espinoza J, Fischer S, et al. Development and performance assessment of a digital serious game to assess multi-patient care skills in a simulated pediatric emergency department. Simul Gaming. 2020;51(4):550–70.
21. Korand S, Fung CC, Cohen S, Talbot TB, Fischer S, Luu C, et al. The association between multitasking and multi-patient care skills in a simulated patient care video game among second year medical students based on specialty choice. Simul Gaming. 2022;53(4):335–52.
22. Chang TP, Hollinger T, Dolby T, Sherman JM. Development and considerations for virtual reality simulations for resuscitation training and stress inoculation. Simul Healthc. 2021;16(6):e219–26.
23. Castillo S, Thomas L, Yarlagadda S, Ahmed Y, Newman JR. Poll everywhere to encourage learner satisfaction and participation in internal medicine fellowship didactics. Cureus. 2020;12(2):e7078.
24. Donkin R, Rasmussen R. Student perception and the effectiveness of Kahoot!: a scoping review in histology, anatomy, and medical education. Anat Sci Educ. 2021;14(5):572–85.
25. Shenson JA, Adams RC, Ahmed ST, Spickard A. Formation of a new entity to support effective use of technology in medical education: the student technology committee. JMIR Med Educ. 2015;1(2):e9. Published 2015 Sep 17.
26. Preiksaitis C, Nash C, Gottlieb M, Chan TM, Alvarez A, Landry A. Brain versus bot: distinguishing letters of recommendation authored by humans compared with artificial intelligence. AEM Educ Train. 2023;7(6). https://doi.org/10.1002/aet2.10924.
27. Sarraf D, Vasiliu V, Imberman B, Lindeman B. Use of artificial intelligence for gender bias analysis in letters of recommendation for general surgery residency candidates. Am J Surg. 2021;222(6):1051–9. https://doi.org/10.1016/j.amjsurg.2021.09.034.

28. Leung TI, Sagar A, Shroff S, Henry TL. Can AI mitigate bias in writing letters of recommendation? JMIR Med Educ. 2023;9:e51494. Published 2023 Aug 23
29. Kaplan DM, Palitsky R, Arconada Alvarez SJ, Pozzo NS, Greenleaf MN, Atkinson CA, et al. What's in a name? Experimental evidence of gender bias in recommendation letters generated by ChatGPT. J Med Internet Res. 2024;26:e51837. Published 2024 Mar 5.
30. Giray L. Prompt engineering with ChatGPT: a guide for academic writers. Ann Biomed Eng. 2023;51(12):2629–33.
31. Kung TH, Cheatham M, Medenilla A, Sillos C, De Leon L, Elepaño C, et al. Performance of ChatGPT on USMLE: potential for AI-assisted medical education using large language models. PLOS Digit Health. 2023;2(2):e0000198.
32. Gilson A, Safranek CW, Huang T, Socrates V, Chi L, Taylor RA, et al. How does ChatGPT perform on the United States medical licensing examination (USMLE)? The implications of large language models for medical education and knowledge assessment. JMIR Med Educ. 2024;10:e57594.
33. Nachshon A, Batzofin B, Beil M, Van Heerden PV. ChatGPT-based learning: generative artificial intelligence in medical education. Med Sci Educ. 2023;33(3):747–58.
34. Reis F, Lenz C, Gossen M, Volk HD, Drzeniek NM. Practical applications of large language models for health care professionals and scientists. JMIR Med Inform. 2024;12:e58478. Published 2024 Sep 5.
35. Khan RA, Jawaid M, Khan AR, Sajjad M. ChatGPT—Reshaping medical education and clinical management. Pak J Med Sci. 2023;39(2):605–7.
36. Keykha A, Behravesh S, Ghaemi F. ChatGPT and medical research: a meta-synthesis of opportunities and challenges. J Adv Med Educ Prof. 2024;12(3):135–47. Published 2024 Jul 1.
37. Gao CA, Howard FM, Markov NS, Dyer EC, Ramesh S, Luo Y, et al. Comparing scientific abstracts generated by ChatGPT to original abstracts using an artificial intelligence output detector, plagiarism detector, and blinded human reviewers. NPJ Digit Med. 2023;6(1):75.
38. Macdonald C, Adeloye D, Sheikh A, Rudan I. Can ChatGPT draft a research article? An example of population-level vaccine effectiveness analysis. J Glob Health. 2023;13:01003. Published 2023 Feb 17.
39. Chen TJ. ChatGPT and other artificial intelligence applications speed up scientific writing. J Chin Med Assoc. 2023;86(4):351–3.
40. Tools such as ChatGPT threaten transparent science; here are our ground rules for their use. Nature. 2023;613(7945):612.
41. Liebrenz M, Schleifer R, Buadze A, Bhugra D, Smith A. Generating scholarly content with ChatGPT: ethical challenges for medical publishing. Lancet Digit Health. 2023;5(3):e105–6.
42. Busch F, Adams LC, Bressem KK. Biomedical ethical aspects towards the implementation of artificial intelligence in medical education. Med Sci Educ. 2023;33(4):1007–12.

Index

T. Adirim (ed.), *Digital Health, AI and Generative AI in Healthcare*,
https://doi.org/10.1007/978-3-031-83526-1

9783031835254